PROTEIN POWDER COOKING

...Beyond the Shake

200 Delicious Recipes to Supercharge Every Dish with Whey, Soy, Casein and More

Courtney Nielsen

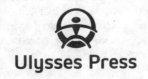

Ulysses Press

Published in the U.S. by
Ulysses Press
P.O. Box 3440
Berkeley, CA 94703
www.ulyssespress.com

ISBN: 978-1-61243-524-4
Library of Congress Control Number: 2015944222

Printed in Canada by Marquis Book Printing
10 9 8 7 6 5 4 3 2 1

Acquisitions Editor: Kelly Reed
Managing Editor: Claire Chun
Editor: Renee Rutledge
Proofreader: Barbara Schultz
Cover design: what!design @ whatweb.com
Cover photos: pancakes © mama_mia/shutterstock.com; measuring scoop ©
    marekuliasz/shutterstock.com; chocolate coconut candy © violeta pasat/
    shutterstock.com; cookie jar © MShev/shutterstock.com; chocolate lava
    cake © comeirrez/shutterstock.com; chocolate and vanilla protein powder ©
    BLACKDAY/shutterstock.com
Interior design: Jake Flaherty

Distributed by Publishers Group West

CONTENTS

INTRODUCTION

Why Use Protein Powder?

It's typical to think of a shaker bottle when you think of protein powder. After all, the most common way to consume protein powder is by simply mixing it with water and drinking it. But think of all the other foods you eat throughout the day. If you could boost their protein content while enhancing their flavor, you could meet your protein needs and health goals while continuing to eat a delicious variety of foods!

A person's protein needs are determined by both their weight and activity level. The bare minimum recommended protein intake in grams is about 0.36 grams per pound of body weight per day. Still, taking in more protein than this can be very helpful for increasing your metabolism, building lean muscle tissue, feeling more satiated by meals, and even boosting your immune system. If you're doing heavy strength or athletic training, your protein needs may be as high as 1 gram of protein per pound of body weight per day.

Choosing a Protein Supplement

When choosing a protein powder, there are three main things to consider: the nutritional label, the quality of the brand, and the protein source.

Nutritionally, I prefer a protein powder that has little or no sugar and very few grams of carbs or fats. This way, I am only adding protein to my recipes, and I can have more control over the nutritional content of each one. In addition, I am always sure to pay attention to the ingredients list, looking for the shortest lists I can find, which usually mean a higher-quality powder.

You can choose a brand by looking for detailed information on the company's website and for reviews of the brand on other websites. I make sure to go with trusted brands that aim for high quality rather than cutting corners just for the sake of price.

Finally, the type of protein itself is going to be a personal choice. The main kinds I would look for are whey or casein (dairy proteins), soy, or a vegan protein blend containing all the essential amino acids. All of these types are interchangeable in each recipe, so it is very easy to make any of the recipes vegan or dairy-free if need be, but you may still need to test various powder types for digestibility and flavor before buying a large quantity. Most companies will send protein powder samples for you to try if you go to their website, and nutrition stores often sell sample sizes as well!

No matter what kind you get, you can measure protein powder using cups or tablespoons, but I find that using a digital scale to weigh your protein is much more precise and effective for baking. For this reason, I include the number of grams of protein powder to include in each recipe as well.

Ingredient Guide

You have your own goals and dietary needs, which means that you may wish to modify some of the recipes in this book. Luckily, most of these recipes can be easily adapted to fit your personal plan.

For those interested in eating more whole grains, feel free to use white whole wheat flour in any recipe containing flour. I have tested each recipe (that contains flour) using 100 percent white whole wheat flour in order to make sure that the taste and texture come out just right. Please note: I used white whole wheat, which is a different variety of the same grain, but has a milder texture and flavor than regular whole wheat and is therefore easier to incorporate into recipes. More like white flour, white whole wheat tends to require less liquid in baking than regular whole wheat, so be sure to take that into account as well.

If you are trying to remove dairy from your diet, any recipe in this book can be made dairy-free by choosing a nondairy milk, yogurt, or cheese, all of which are becoming increasingly available at local grocery stores and can taste just as good!

The same goes for sugar. If I call for sugar in a recipe, feel free to sub out some or all of it for agave, baking stevia, or erythritol unless otherwise noted.

If a recipe is gluten-free and calls for flours you don't normally use, it is often possible to use regular flour instead. However, many of the recipes in this book use ground flaxseed. Its specific structure allows for better texture in protein powder recipes. You can often buy this in bulk (to make it more cost-effective) and use it in all kinds of recipes! I swear by it, and think it should be a staple for anyone looking to bake healthfully and with protein powder!

Finally, a note on protein powder flavor, especially for those looking to buy only one or two kinds. If you only want to bake the sweets, at the very least, get vanilla protein powder. If you want to make only savory items, you'll only need the plain. But if you want to be able to make any recipe in this book, definitely invest in at least a tub each of vanilla and plain. Beyond that, there are numerous flavors of protein powders. I would also suggest getting a chocolate protein powder, but if you know there is a flavor you love, buy that too, as you can use the flavored powders to elevate the flavor of your recipes even more! Strawberry, cinnamon, mocha, banana, cake batter, and pumpkin pie are some of the flavors I've used in my baking, and I think they are definitely worth a try!

Tools to Have Handy

- Blender
- Bowls (small, medium, and large)
- Digital scale
- Food processor
- Measuring cups
- Measuring spoons
- Muffin pan and/or doughnut pan
- Various baking sheets and cake pans
- Whisks

A Note about the Calorie Calculations

To ensure uniformity, all recipe nutritional facts are calculated using unsweetened almond milk for "milk," nonfat plain Greek yogurt for "Greek yogurt," whole wheat flour for "flour," and Isopure protein powder for "protein powder." Also note that "oil" refers to coconut or canola oil, which are interchangeable, and all butter used throughout the book is unsalted.

BREAKFAST BOWLS

Taking a different route from cold cereal in the morning can be fun—and more nutritious! Of course you'll have new flavors and textures to enjoy, but you'll also cut down on unhealthy processed foods while getting more of the whole foods your body thrives on. Some of these recipes combine different fruits and protein powders to make thick smoothie bowls. The other ones are hot breakfast bowls that will really fill you up. Either way they are all simple to make and encourage you to get creative with healthy toppings!

ACAI BOWL

¼ cup (30 grams) vanilla protein powder

¼ cup milk

⅓ cup acai juice

1 cup mixed frozen berries

¼ cup Greek yogurt

1 teaspoon acai powder

2 tablespoons chia seeds, to top

¼ cup fresh blueberries, to top

Combine all of the ingredients except the toppings together in a blender until smooth. Pour into a bowl and decorate with toppings. Enjoy immediately!

MAKES 1 SERVING

NUTRITION PER SERVING				
280 calories	3 g fat	33 g carbs	9 g fiber	34 g protein

CRUNCHY PEACH BOWL

¼ cup (30 grams) vanilla protein powder

¼ cup orange juice

⅓ cup milk

1 cup frozen sliced peaches

¼ cup Greek yogurt

1 tablespoon ground flaxseed

1 teaspoon powdered ginger, to top

¼ cup granola, to top

Combine all of the ingredients except the toppings together in a blender until smooth. Pour into a bowl and decorate with toppings. Enjoy immediately!

MAKES 1 SERVING

NUTRITION PER SERVING				
301 calories	3 g fat	33 g carbs	6 g fiber	37 g protein

STRAWBERRY BANANA BOWL

¼ cup (30 grams) vanilla or
   strawberry protein powder

¼ cup orange juice

⅓ cup milk

½ cup chopped frozen strawberries

½ cup chopped frozen bananas

¼ cup Greek yogurt

½ cup chopped fresh strawberries,
   to top

2 tablespoons slivered almonds, to
   top

Combine all of the ingredients except the toppings together in a blender until smooth. Pour into a bowl and decorate with toppings. Enjoy immediately!

MAKES 1 SERVING

NUTRITION PER SERVING				
275 calories	1 g fat	33 g carbs	4 g fiber	34 g protein

ZINGER BOWL

¼ cup (30 grams) vanilla protein powder

⅓ cup orange juice

¼ cup milk

½ cup sliced frozen kiwi

½ cup frozen berries

¼ cup Greek yogurt

1 tablespoon ground flaxseed

2 tablespoons shredded dried coconut, to top

¼ cup any fruit (like chopped mango or berries), to top

Combine all of the ingredients except the toppings together in a blender until smooth. Pour into a bowl and decorate with toppings. Enjoy immediately!

MAKES 1 SERVING

NUTRITION PER SERVING				
297 calories	4 g fat	31 g carbs	7 g fiber	35 g protein

MANGO SUNRISE BOWL

¼ cup (30 grams) vanilla protein powder

⅓ cup orange juice

¼ cup milk

1 cup chopped mango

⅓ cup Greek yogurt or cottage cheese

1 tablespoon ground chia or flaxseed

2 tablespoons chia seeds, to top

¼ cup granola, to top

Combine all of the ingredients except the toppings together in a blender until smooth. Pour into a bowl and decorate with toppings. Enjoy immediately!

MAKES 1 SERVING

NUTRITION PER SERVING				
337 calories	4 g fat	39 g carbs	5 g fiber	37 g protein

FRUIT SALAD FOR TWO

¼ cup (30 grams) vanilla protein powder

¾ cup Greek yogurt

2 cups of your favorite chopped fruits

2 tablespoons chopped nuts, to top

2 tablespoons chia or flaxseeds, to top

3 tablespoons granola, to top

1 Combine vanilla protein powder and Greek yogurt in a bowl. Add the chopped fruits. Mix to combine well.

2 Divide into two bowls and add toppings. Enjoy immediately!

MAKES 2 SERVINGS

NUTRITION PER SERVING				
153 calories	0 g fat	15 g carbs	2 g fiber	22 g protein

BANANA OATMEAL

½ cup rolled oats

1 cup any milk or water

3 tablespoons (20 grams) vanilla or
banana protein powder

½ large banana, chopped

1 tablespoon chia or flaxseeds

1 Combine oats and milk or water in a microwave-safe bowl or small pot. In the microwave or on the stovetop, cook the oats until they have absorbed most of the liquid and are cooked through.

2 Add more liquid if necessary to cook the oats fully without drying them out.

3 Add the remaining ingredients, stir well, and enjoy.

MAKES 1 SERVING

NUTRITION PER SERVING				
368 calories	5 g fat	61 g carbs	8 g fiber	28 g protein

OVERNIGHT CREAMY OATMEAL

3 tablespoons (20 grams) vanilla or other protein powder

½ cup rolled oats

½ cup milk or water

¼ cup Greek yogurt

½ cup your choice of chopped fruit, to top

2 tablespoons chopped nuts, to top

2 tablespoons chia or flaxseeds, to top

3 tablespoons granola, to top

2 teaspoons peanut butter, to top

1 Combine all of the ingredients except the toppings in a sealable container. Refrigerator overnight.

2 In the morning, stir the oats again, add the toppings, and enjoy.

MAKES 1 SERVING

NUTRITION PER SERVING				
258 calories	3 g fat	30 g carbs	3 g fiber	31 g protein

BERRY NUT OATMEAL

½ cup rolled oats

1 cup any milk or water

3 tablespoons (20 grams) vanilla
protein powder

1 cup your choice of fresh berries

¼ teaspoon almond extract (optional)

2 tablespoons chopped almonds,
walnuts, or pecans

1 Combine oats and any milk or water in a microwave-safe bowl or
small pot. In the microwave or on the stovetop, cook the oats until
they have absorbed most of the liquid and are cooked through. Add
more liquid if necessary to cook the oats fully without drying them
out.

2 Add the remaining ingredients, stir well, and enjoy.

MAKES 1 SERVING

NUTRITION PER SERVING				
418 calories	13 g fat	44 g carbs	7 g fiber	34 g protein

QUINOA PB CUP BREAKFAST BOWL FOR TWO

⅓ cup uncooked quinoa, rinsed

1 cup any milk or water

3 tablespoons (20 grams) chocolate protein

1 tablespoon peanut butter, to top

2 teaspoons cocoa powder, to top

1 In a covered pot or pan, simmer the quinoa in the milk or water for 20 minutes, or cook fully in a rice cooker until fluffy.

2 Combine cooked quinoa with protein powder and add toppings.

MAKES 2 SERVINGS

NUTRITION PER SERVING				
199 calories	6 g fat	30 g carbs	3 g fiber	16 g protein

ALMOND APRICOT HOT GRAINS BOWL

If you cook up a whole grain like quinoa ahead of time, you can use it to make quick, healthy meals all week. This recipe is a tasty way to use a pre-cooked grain for breakfast.

½ cup cooked quinoa or other whole grain

½ cup any milk

3 tablespoons (20 grams) vanilla protein powder

3 dried apricots, chopped

2 tablespoons slivered almonds

¼ teaspoon almond extract (optional)

1 Combine cooked grains and milk in a microwave-safe bowl. In the microwave, cook grains until they are heated through.

2 Add the other ingredients, stir well, and enjoy.

MAKES 1 SERVING

NUTRITION PER SERVING				
366 calories	10 g fat	38 g carbs	6 g fiber	28 g protein

SMOOTHIES

Smoothies are wonderful because you can make them quickly anytime you need them, and there are so many ways to do them! The ones in this chapter are made to fit all kinds of tastes and are all extremely nutritious in different ways. Each smoothie recipe is great for one meal or two snacks!

CHOCOLATE-COVERED BERRY SMOOTHIE

Having chocolate and berries in the same glass for breakfast squashes my morning sweet tooth, plus it's great for pre- or post-workout nutrition.

¼ cup (30 grams) chocolate protein

1 cup milk

1 tablespoon ground flaxseed

1 cup mixed frozen berries

⅓ cup Greek yogurt

Blend all of the ingredients in a blender. Enjoy immediately!

MAKES 1 SMOOTHIE | GLUTEN-FREE

NUTRITION PER SMOOTHIE				
317 calories	7 g fat	30 g carbs	12 g fiber	37 g protein

PB AND J SMOOTHIE

PB and J is not just for the kids. I love peanut butter and jelly anything, and smoothies are a really healthy way to get that flavor combo!

¼ cup (30 grams) vanilla protein powder

1 cup milk

1 tablespoon ground flaxseed

⅔ cup frozen berries

½ sliced frozen banana

1 tablespoon peanut butter

⅓ cup Greek yogurt

Blend all of the ingredients in a blender. Enjoy immediately!

MAKES 1 SMOOTHIE | GLUTEN-FREE

NUTRITION PER SMOOTHIE				
420 calories	13 g fat	36 g carbs	8 g fiber	41 g protein

CHOCOLATE PB CUP SMOOTHIE CUP

When you really want something dessert-like, it's not a bad idea to satisfy the craving with a healthy smoothie! The taste and texture in this one are on-point, and it's really good for you!

¼ cup (30 grams) chocolate protein

1 cup milk

2 tablespoons cocoa powder

1 tablespoon peanut butter

1 tablespoon ground flaxseed

¼ cup pumpkin puree

Blend all of the ingredients in a blender. Enjoy immediately!

MAKES 1 SMOOTHIE | GLUTEN-FREE

NUTRITION PER SMOOTHIE				
367 calories	15 g fat	22 g carbs	10 g fiber	43 g protein

PUMPKIN PIE SMOOTH...

I don't wait for fall on this one; a Pumpkin Pie Smoothie is actually really
to have any time of the year! Just think about all the vitamin A you'll get, too

- ¼ cup (30 grams) vanilla protein powder
- ½ cup milk
- ½ cup carrot juice
- ¼ cup pumpkin puree

- 1 teaspoon grated fresh ginger *or* ½ teaspoon ground ginger
- ½ teaspoon ground cinnamon
- ½ sliced frozen banana

Blend all of the ingredients in a blender. Enjoy immediately!

MAKES 1 SMOOTHIE | GLUTEN-FREE

NUTRITION PER SMOOTHIE				
255 calories	3 g fat	25 g carbs	5 g fiber	33 g protein

Tip: Instead of grating fresh ginger every time, you can grate it ahead and freeze with water in an ice cube tray, then store in a freezer bag!

NGE DREAMSICLE
SMOOTHIE

...ith your protein-packed breakfast can go a long way
goals. This amazingly delicious smoothie could be

¼ cup (30 grams) vanilla protein powder

½ cup orange juice

½ cup milk

½ cup sliced frozen peaches

½ sliced frozen banana

⅓ cup Greek yogurt

Blend all of the ingredients in a blender. Enjoy immediately!

MAKES 1 SMOOTHIE | GLUTEN-FREE

NUTRITION PER SMOOTHIE				
346 calories	2 g fat	49 g carbs	5 g fiber	37 g protein

PEACHY KEEN SMOOTHIE

With all the different nutrition-packed ingredients in this smoothie, it really is a breakfast of champions! I definitely recommend slicing and freezing your own fresh kiwi to make this one!

¼ cup (30 grams) vanilla protein powder

1 cup orange juice

½ cup sliced frozen kiwi

½ cup sliced frozen peaches

⅓ cup Greek yogurt

1 tablespoon ground flaxseed

1 teaspoon grated fresh or frozen ginger *or* ½ teaspoon ground ginger

Blend all of the ingredients in a blender. Enjoy immediately!

MAKES 1 SMOOTHIE | GLUTEN-FREE

NUTRITION PER SMOOTHIE				
445 calories	4 g fat	63 g carbs	8 g fiber	44 g protein

Tip: Instead of grating fresh ginger every time, you can grate it ahead and freeze with water in an ice cube tray, then store in a freezer bag!

BERRY ZINGER SMOOTHIE

This smoothie has a very zesty flavor that always helps me wake up or feel refreshed. Plus, cinnamon is great for keeping that metabolism and immune system revved up!

- ¼ cup (30 grams) vanilla protein powder
- 1 cup orange juice
- ½ cup sliced frozen kiwi
- ½ cup frozen berries
- ⅓ cup Greek yogurt
- ½ teaspoon ground cinnamon

Blend all of the ingredients in a blender. Enjoy immediately!

MAKES 1 SMOOTHIE | GLUTEN-FREE

NUTRITION PER SMOOTHIE				
375 calories	1 g fat	52 g carbs	5 g fiber	41 g protein

JAVA CAPPUCCINO SMOOTHIE

I say ditch the coffee shop habit and start throwing these together in the morning instead. They are delicious but much healthier, and you get to skip waiting in line!

¼ cup (30 grams) vanilla or chocolate protein powder

½ cup brewed coffee or espresso

½ cup milk

1 cup ice

⅓ cup Greek yogurt

1 tablespoon instant coffee or espresso powder

Blend all of the ingredients in a blender. Enjoy immediately!

MAKES 1 SMOOTHIE | GLUTEN-FREE

NUTRITION PER SMOOTHIE				
204 calories	3 g fat	6 g carbs	1 g fiber	39 g protein

CINNAMON OATMEAL SMOOTHIE

This smoothie is extra well rounded, with slower-digesting carbs from the rolled oats that can help keep you full longer when combined with the protein. Be sure to buy gluten-free, certified oats if you need this to be gluten-free.

¼ cup (30 grams) vanilla or cinnamon protein powder

1 cup milk

½ cup ice

¼ cup rolled oats

⅓ cup Greek yogurt or cottage cheese

½ teaspoon ground cinnamon

Blend all of the ingredients in a blender. Enjoy immediately!

MAKES 1 SMOOTHIE | GLUTEN-FREE

NUTRITION PER SMOOTHIE				
256 calories	4 g fat	63 g carbs	8 g fiber	44 g protein

SUNRISE STRAWBERRY SMOOTHIE

There is some serious fruit flavor going on in this smoothie. It is really refreshing and tasty for any time of the day!

¼ cup (30 grams) vanilla or strawberry protein powder

½ cup orange juice

½ cup milk

½ cup chopped frozen strawberries

½ cup chopped frozen chopped bananas

⅓ cup Greek yogurt

Blend all of the ingredients in a blender. Enjoy immediately!

MAKES 1 SMOOTHIE | GLUTEN-FREE

NUTRITION PER SMOOTHIE				
327 calories	2 g fat	44 g carbs	5 g fiber	35 g protein

PIÑA COLADA SMOOTHIE

If I had to choose just one smoothie above all other smoothies, it would be this one. I just can't get enough of it!

¼ cup (30 grams) vanilla protein powder

½ cup pineapple juice

½ cup coconut milk

½ cup chopped frozen pineapple

½ teaspoon coconut extract

½ cup ice

⅓ cup Greek yogurt or cottage cheese

Blend all of the ingredients in a blender. Enjoy immediately!

MAKES 1 SMOOTHIE | GLUTEN-FREE

NUTRITION PER SMOOTHIE				
282 calories	3 g fat	30 g carbs	2 g fiber	34 g protein

MOCHA SMOOTHIE

Tasty with a wake-me-up effect, I love to grab this smoothie before starting my day!

⅓ cup (40 grams) chocolate protein powder

1 cup milk

½ cup ice

1 tablespoon cocoa powder

1 tablespoon almond butter

2 tablespoons instant coffee or espresso powder

Blend all of the ingredients in a blender. Enjoy immediately!

MAKES 1 SMOOTHIE | GLUTEN-FREE

NUTRITION PER SMOOTHIE				
356 calories	14 g fat	16 g carbs	5 g fiber	46 g protein

POWERFUL PINEAPPLE SMOOTHIE

This is a great alternative to the Piña Colada Smoothie if you aren't a fan of coconut, plus it has the added benefit of omega-3s and fiber from the chia or flaxseed.

¼ cup (30 grams) vanilla protein powder

½ cup pineapple juice

½ cup milk

½ cup frozen, chopped pineapple

2 tablespoons ground chia or flaxseed

⅓ cup Greek yogurt or cottage cheese

Blend all of the ingredients in a blender. Enjoy immediately!

MAKES 1 SMOOTHIE | GLUTEN-FREE

NUTRITION PER SMOOTHIE				
373 calories	7 g fat	36 g carbs	6 g fiber	39 g protein

PEACHES AND CREAM SMOOTHIE

This sweet treat reminds me of a summer afternoon when the peaches are just becoming ripe. Strawberries add sweetness and color to the smoothie!

¼ cup (30 grams) vanilla protein powder

½ cup apple juice

½ cup milk

½ cup chopped frozen peaches

½ cup chopped frozen strawberries

⅓ cup Greek yogurt or cottage cheese

Blend all of the ingredients in a blender. Enjoy immediately!

MAKES 1 SMOOTHIE | GLUTEN-FREE

NUTRITION PER SMOOTHIE				
293 calories	1 g fat	33 g carbs	3 g fiber	36 g protein

THE GREEN BANANA SMOOTHIE

Healthy fat from the avocado, which can be fresh or frozen, and the added nutrition from the spirulina (or matcha green tea powder) makes this smoothie a great breakfast that tastes like a banana milkshake!

- ¼ cup (30 grams) vanilla or banana protein powder
- 1 cup milk
- ⅔ cup chopped frozen banana
- ⅓ cup chopped avocado
- 2 teaspoons spirulina powder

Blend all of the ingredients in a blender. Enjoy immediately!

MAKES 1 SMOOTHIE | GLUTEN-FREE

NUTRITION PER SMOOTHIE				
386 calories	14 g fat	32 g carbs	8 g fiber	33 g protein

BANANA CREAM PIE SMOOTHIE

If you're a banana lover like me, sometimes all you need is a straight-up banana smoothie. The best thing about banana is really the ice cream–like feel it has when frozen and then blended—so the smoothie is more like a creamy milkshake!

⅓ cup (40 grams) vanilla, banana, or peanut butter protein powder

1 cup milk

⅔ cup chopped frozen bananas

⅓ cup ice

⅓ cup Greek yogurt or cottage cheese

Blend all of the ingredients in a blender. Enjoy immediately!

MAKES 1 SMOOTHIE | GLUTEN-FREE

NUTRITION PER SMOOTHIE				
317 calories	3 g fat	26 g carbs	3 g fiber	45 g protein

BERRY SUPER SMOOTHIE

With all the antioxidants packed into this smoothie, it really is a super shake! If you can find the goji or acai powder, I think it is definitely worth a try.

¼ cup (30 grams) vanilla or berry protein powder

½ cup milk

½ cup acai or pomegranate juice

½ cup frozen blueberries

½ cup frozen raspberries

1 tablespoon goji or acai powder

1 tablespoon ground chia or flaxseed

Blend all of the ingredients in a blender. Enjoy immediately!

MAKES 1 SMOOTHIE | GLUTEN-FREE

NUTRITION PER SMOOTHIE				
375 calories	6 g fat	40 g carbs	10 g fiber	38 g protein

GREEN DREAM SMOOTHIE

If you've been meaning to add more greens to your diet, but aren't so into salads or just want something on the go, try throwing them into a creamy and zesty smoothie like this one.

⅓ cup (40 grams) vanilla protein powder

½ cup orange juice

½ cup milk

1 cup baby spinach leaves

⅓ cup chopped frozen avocado

2 tablespoons rolled oats or ground chia or flaxseed

Blend all of the ingredients in a blender. Enjoy immediately!

MAKES 1 SMOOTHIE | GLUTEN-FREE

NUTRITION PER SMOOTHIE				
402 calories	16 g fat	23 g carbs	9 g fiber	42 g protein

CREAMY MATCHA SMOOTHIE

I was inspired by the matcha Frappuccinos at Starbucks to whip up this one. Having a bag of matcha powder handy makes it really easy and delicious to get more healthy and slimming green tea into your day! Feel free to substitute the banana with a small chopped peach instead.

¼ cup (30 grams) vanilla protein powder

1 cup milk

½ cup chopped frozen banana

½ cup ice

⅓ cup Greek yogurt or cottage cheese

2 tablespoons matcha green tea powder

Blend all of the ingredients in a blender. Enjoy immediately!

MAKES 1 SMOOTHIE | GLUTEN-FREE

NUTRITION PER SMOOTHIE				
312 calories	4 g fat	63 g carbs	8 g fiber	44 g protein

CANTALOUPE DELIGHT SMOOTHIE

It's probably time to get yourself a cantaloupe-based smoothie if you haven't done so yet. It can be fresh or frozen, but make sure you use a very sweet and ripe one before you freeze it or use it in your smoothie.

¼ cup (30 grams) vanilla protein powder

½ cup apple juice

½ cup milk

1 cup chopped cantaloupe

⅓ cup Greek yogurt or cottage cheese

2 tablespoons ground chia or flaxseed

Blend all of the ingredients in a blender. Enjoy immediately!

MAKES 1 SMOOTHIE | GLUTEN-FREE

NUTRITION PER SMOOTHIE				
372 calories	8 g fat	38 g carbs	6 g fiber	39 g protein

PANCAKES AND WAFFLES

I tend to have a sweet tooth first thing in the morning, so I gravitate toward waffles, pancakes, and crepes for breakfast. Occasionally, I'll even want some for dinner! Each one of these recipes is very easy to make and as soft and fluffy as can be. There is something for everyone in this section, whether you want traditional, low-carb, or even something wild—like banana-bacon pancakes!

CHOCOLATE BANANA WAFFLES

⅓ cup (40 grams) vanilla protein powder

1 large banana

1 egg

2 tablespoons cocoa powder

2 tablespoons agave syrup

2 tablespoons coconut oil

½ cup flour

1 teaspoon baking soda

1 Preheat the waffle iron.

2 Mix all of the ingredients together.

3 Scoop the batter in fourths into the four sides of the waffle iron. Close the lid and wait for 2 to 3 minutes or until you can smell the waffles and steam begins to escape from the waffle iron.

4 Carefully lift the lid and make sure the waffle has begun to brown before removing the waffles.

MAKES 4 SERVINGS

NUTRITION PER SERVING				
238 calories	8 g fat	27 g carbs	3 g fiber	14 g protein

SUPER WAFFLES

¼ cup (30 grams) any flavor protein
   powder

1 egg

¼ cup liquid egg whites

3 tablespoons Greek yogurt

2 tablespoons ground flaxseed

1 Preheat the waffle iron.

2 Mix all of the ingredients together.

3 Scoop the batter in fourths into the four sides of the waffle iron. Close
the lid and wait for 2 to 3 minutes or until you can smell the waffles
and steam begins to escape from the waffle iron.

4 Carefully lift the lid and make sure the waffle has begun to brown
before removing the waffles.

MAKES 2 SERVINGS | LOW-CARB | GLUTEN-FREE

NUTRITION PER SERVING				
170 calories	7 g fat	5 g carbs	2 g fiber	23 g protein

CHOCOLATE CHIP CAKE WAFFLES

1 cup flour

1 teaspoon baking powder

½ teaspoon baking soda

¼ teaspoon salt

1 egg

½ cup applesauce

½ cup milk

¼ cup (30 grams) vanilla protein powder

1 teaspoon vanilla extract

1 tablespoon coconut oil, melted

2 tablespoons mini chocolate chips

1 Preheat the waffle iron.

2 Mix the first four ingredients together. Add the remaining ingredients, in order, and mix to combine.

3 Scoop one-third of the batter into the waffle iron. Close the lid and wait for 2 to 3 minutes or until you can smell the waffles and steam begins to escape from the waffle iron.

4 Carefully lift the lid and make sure the waffle has begun to brown before removing the waffle and repeating two more times with the remaining batter.

MAKES 3 SERVINGS

NUTRITION PER SERVING				
303 calories	11 g fat	41 g carbs	6 g fiber	14 g protein

ORANGE WALNUT WAFFLES

¼ cup (30 grams) vanilla protein powder

1 cup flour

1 teaspoon baking powder

½ teaspoon baking soda

¼ teaspoon salt

3 tablespoons Greek yogurt

1 tablespoon ground flaxseed

1 tablespoon oil

⅓ cup orange juice

⅔ cup applesauce

2 tablespoons almond any milk

1 Preheat the waffle iron.

2 Mix all of the ingredients together.

3 Scoop the batter in fourths into the four sides of the waffle iron. Close the lid and wait for 2 to 3 minutes or until you can smell the waffles and steam begins to escape from the waffle iron.

4 Carefully lift the lid and make sure the waffle has begun to brown before removing the waffles.

MAKES 4 SERVINGS

NUTRITION PER SERVING				
238 calories	8 g fat	27 g carbs	3 g fiber	14 g protein

MAPLE WAFFLES

¼ cup (30 grams) vanilla protein powder

1 cup flour

1 teaspoon baking powder

½ teaspoon baking soda

2 tablespoons coconut oil

¼ teaspoon maple extract or ½ teaspoon vanilla extract

2 tablespoons maple syrup

2 tablespoons Greek yogurt

½ cup milk, or more as necessary

1 Preheat the waffle iron.

2 Mix all of the ingredients together.

3 Scoop the batter in fourths into the four sides of the waffle iron. Close the lid and wait for 2 to 3 minutes or until you can smell the waffles and steam begins to escape from the waffle iron.

4 Carefully lift the lid and make sure the waffle has begun to brown before removing the waffles.

MAKES 4 SERVINGS

NUTRITION PER SERVING				
238 calories	8 g fat	27 g carbs	3 g fiber	14 g protein

CHEESY CHIVE WAFFLES

⅓ cup (40 grams) plain protein powder

2 tablespoons ground flaxseed

1 egg

5 tablespoons liquid egg whites

3 tablespoons shredded cheese (cheddar or your favorite!)

2 tablespoons Greek yogurt

2 tablespoons chopped chives or green onions

2 tablespoons water or milk

¼ teaspoon garlic powder

⅛ teaspoon salt

1 Preheat the waffle iron.

2 Mix all of the ingredients together.

3 Scoop the batter in fourths into the four sides of the waffle iron. Close the lid and wait for 2 to 3 minutes or until you can smell the waffles and steam begins to escape from the waffle iron.

4 Carefully lift the lid and make sure the waffle has begun to brown before removing the waffles.

MAKES 2 SERVINGS | LOW-CARB | GLUTEN-FREE

NUTRITION PER SERVING				
223 calories	10 g fat	3 g carbs	2 g fiber	30 g protein

PERFECT PANCAKES

¼ cup liquid egg whites

2 tablespoons ground flaxseed

3 to 4 tablespoons (26 grams) of your favorite protein powder

2 tablespoons Greek yogurt

1 Preheat a pan over medium heat and coat with cooking spray, or (my favorite) add 1 teaspoon extra-virgin coconut oil to the pan.

2 Whisk all of the ingredients together well and add 1 tablespoon of water at a time until you have a semi-thick pancake batter.

3 When the pan is hot, spoon out a couple of tablespoons to make small pancakes. I like to make 3 or 4 small pancakes!

MAKES 1 SERVING | LOW-CARB | GLUTEN-FREE

NUTRITION PER SERVING				
188 calories	5 g fat	7 g carbs	6 g fiber	28 g protein

BANANA BACON FRITTERS

1 cup (110 grams) vanilla, cinnamon, peanut butter protein powder

3 bananas

1½ cups oats

2 eggs

½ teaspoon baking powder

8 pieces crispy, cooked turkey or vegan bacon, finely chopped

1 Preheat a pan over medium heat and coat with cooking spray, or (my favorite) add 1 teaspoon (5 grams) extra-virgin coconut oil to the pan.

2 Whisk all of the ingredients together well until you have a thick pancake batter.

3 When the pan is hot, spoon out a couple of tablespoons to make small pancakes. Cook on both sides and serve hot!

MAKES 4 SERVINGS

NUTRITION PER SERVING				
238 calories	8 g fat	27 g carbs	3 g fiber	14 g protein

VANILLA CREPES

½ cup plus 3 tablespoons liquid egg whites

⅓ cup (40 grams) vanilla protein powder

2 tablespoons coconut flour

2½ tablespoons ground flaxseed

1 tablespoon oil

1 tablespoon brown sugar

1 Preheat a pan over medium heat and coat with cooking spray, or (my favorite) add 1 teaspoon extra-virgin coconut oil to the pan.

2 Whisk all of the ingredients together well until you have what looks like a thin pancake batter.

3 When the pan is hot, pour enough onto the pan to make a thin, even layer. Tilt the pan to make sure it is even. Cook for a minute or two, until you can flip the crepe, and finish cooking.

4 Serve plain or rolled around fruit or other toppings!

MAKES 2 SERVINGS

NUTRITION PER SERVING				
289 calories	12 g fat	14 g carbs	5 g fiber	31 g protein

SWEET POTATO PANCAKES

⅓ cup (40 grams) vanilla, cinnamon, or maple protein powder

¼ cup baked, mashed (or pureed) sweet potato *or* pumpkin

2 tablespoons Greek yogurt or cottage cheese

1 tablespoon liquid egg whites

⅓ cup oats

1 tablespoon coconut flour

½ teaspoon ground cinnamon

pinch of nutmeg

½ teaspoon baking powder

¼ teaspoon baking soda

3 to 4-plus tablespoons water

1 Throw everything into a blender or food processor until well blended.

2 Heat a pancake griddle to medium heat, and make sure it's ready by dripping a little water on it to see if it sizzles.

3 Spray the griddle with cooking spray, and scoop pancakes on the pan 2 tablespoons at a time (I just use a ¼ measuring cup and pour half of it out.) If the griddle is the right temperature, about 30 seconds per side should be about right, but watch closely!

4 Serve hot, with some berry compote (just heat up ¼ cup frozen berries), a little light agave syrup (my suggestion would be a good calorie-reduced version), or a bit of light aerosol whipped cream.

MAKES 1 SERVING

NUTRITION PER SERVING				
351 calories	37 g fat	6 g carbs	0 g fiber	39 g protein

STRAWBERRY CAKE WAFFLES

½ cup (55 grams) vanilla or strawberry protein powder

1 large banana

2 tablespoons brown sugar

⅓ cup milk

6 tablespoons liquid egg whites

1 tablespoon lemon juice

1 tablespoon oil

¼ cup ground flaxseed

½ cup flour

¾ teaspoon baking soda

½ cup chopped fresh strawberries

1 Preheat the waffle iron.

2 Mix all of the ingredients together.

3 Scoop the batter in fourths into the four sides of the waffle iron. Close the lid and wait for 2 to 3 minutes or until you can smell the waffles and steam begins to escape from the waffle iron.

4 Carefully lift the lid and make sure the waffle has begun to brown before removing the waffles.

MAKES 4 SERVINGS

NUTRITION PER SERVING				
238 calories	8 g fat	27 g carbs	3 g fiber	14 g protein

FAT BLUEBERRY PANCAKES

¼ cup (30 grams) vanilla protein powder

3 tablespoons Greek yogurt

⅓ cup liquid egg whites

1 tablespoon ground flaxseed

½ lemon, zested

1 teaspoon honey

¼ cup fresh or frozen blueberries

1 Preheat a pan over medium heat and coat with cooking spray, or (my favorite) add 1 teaspoon (5 grams) extra-virgin coconut oil to the pan.

2 Whisk all of the ingredients except the blueberries together well until you have a thick pancake batter. Stir in the blueberries.

3 When the pan is hot, spoon out a couple of tablespoons at a time to make small pancakes. Cook on both sides, and serve hot!

MAKES 1 SERVING | GLUTEN-FREE

NUTRITION PER SERVING				
260 calories	3 g fat	15 g carbs	3 g fiber	41 g protein

CHUNKY MONKEY PANCAKES

3 bananas

1½ cups oats

1 cup (110 grams) vanilla protein
powder

2 eggs

½ teaspoon baking powder

¼ cup chopped walnuts

1 piece chopped Fudgy Black
Bean Brownie (page 209) or
2 tablespoons chocolate chips

1 Preheat a pan over medium heat and coat with cooking spray, or (my favorite) add 1 teaspoon (5 grams) extra-virgin coconut oil to the pan.

2 Whisk or blend all of the ingredients together well, making sure no banana chunks remain.

3 When the pan is hot, spoon out a couple of tablespoons at a time to make small pancakes. Cook on both sides, and serve hot!

MAKES 4 SERVINGS

NUTRITION PER SERVING				
238 calories	8 g fat	27 g carbs	3 g fiber	16 g protein

FRENCH TOAST

French toast is usually one of the highest-calorie items on any breakfast menu because of the excessive fat in the batter and the sugar that goes on top. But by using egg whites instead of whole eggs, and protein powder for a little sweetness, it's possible to make any kind of French toast healthier! My favorite way to make these is with my homemade Sandwich Bread (page 114) and using calorie-free Walden Farms Pancake Syrup instead of maple syrup.

Tip: Make protein pancakes with any leftover French toast batter by adding a bit of ground flaxseed to thicken, and cook the same way you would other pancakes!

CINNAMON FRENCH TOAST

3 heaping tablespoons (20 grams)
vanilla or cinnamon protein
powder

¼ cup liquid egg whites

½ teaspoon ground cinnamon, plus
more for drizzling (optional)

1 teaspoon maple syrup, plus more
for drizzling

1 large or 2 small, thick slices bread

1 Preheat a large pan over medium heat. Spray with a coat of cooking spray.

2 Mix all but the last ingredient together in a wide bowl.

3 Soak the bread for a few minutes, making sure that there are no dry parts left, and place in the preheated pan.

4 Cook the French toast for a minute or two per side. Top with maple syrup and more cinnamon, if you like!

MAKES 1 SERVING

NUTRITION PER SERVING (batter only)				
133 calories	0 g fat	5 g carbs	0 g fiber	26 g protein

PARIS, FRANCE TOAST

3 heaping tablespoons (20 grams) vanilla protein powder

¼ cup liquid egg whites

½ teaspoon ground cinnamon

1 large or 2 small, thick slices bread

2 tablespoons crème fraîche, to top

2 teaspoons (4 grams) vanilla protein powder, to top

1 Preheat a large pan over medium heat. Spray with a coat of cooking spray.

2 Mix the protein powder, egg whites, and cinnamon together in a wide bowl.

3 Soak the bread for a few minutes, making sure that there are no dry parts left, and place in the preheated pan.

4 Cook the French toast for a minute or two per side. Top with crème fraîche mixed with protein powder.

MAKES 1 SERVING

NUTRITION PER SERVING (batter only)				
133 calories	0 g fat	5 g carbs	0 g fiber	26 g protein

CHOCOLATE FRENCH TOAST

3 heaping tablespoons (20 grams)
  chocolate protein powder

¼ cup liquid egg whites

1 teaspoon cocoa powder

1 teaspoon agave syrup

1 large or 2 small, thick slices bread

2 to 3 tablespoons light whipped
  cream, to top (optional)

1 Preheat a large pan over medium heat. Spray with a coat of cooking spray.

2 Mix the protein powder, egg whites, cocoa powder, and agave syrup together in a wide bowl.

3 Soak the bread for a few minutes, making sure that there are no dry parts left, and place in the preheated pan.

4 Cook the French toast for a minute or two per side. Top with whipped cream, if you like.

MAKES 1 SERVING

NUTRITION PER SERVING (batter only)				
133 calories	0 g fat	5 g carbs	0 g fiber	26 g protein

VANILLA BEAN FRENCH TOAST

3 heaping tablespoons (20 grams) vanilla protein powder

¼ cup liquid egg whites

½ teaspoon vanilla bean paste

1 teaspoon maple syrup

1 large or 2 small, thick slices bread

2 to 3 tablespoons light whipped cream, to top (optional)

1 Preheat a large pan over medium heat. Spray with a coat of cooking spray.

2 Mix the protein powder, egg whites, vanilla bean paste, and maple syrup together in a wide bowl.

3 Soak the bread for a few minutes, making sure that there are no dry parts left, and place in the preheated pan.

4 Cook the French toast for a minute or two per side. Top with whipped cream, if you like.

MAKES 1 SERVING

NUTRITION PER SERVING (batter only)				
133 calories	0 g fat	5 g carbs	0 g fiber	26 g protein

STRAWBERRIES AND CREAM FRENCH TOAST

3 heaping tablespoons (20 grams) strawberry protein powder

¼ cup liquid egg whites

1 teaspoon strawberry jelly

1 large or 2 small, thick slices bread

2 to 3 tablespoons light whipped cream, to top (optional)

1 Preheat a large pan over medium heat. Spray with a coat of cooking spray.

2 Mix the protein powder, egg whites, and strawberry jelly together in a wide bowl.

3 Soak the bread for a few minutes, making sure that there are no dry parts left, and place in the preheated pan.

4 Cook the French toast for a minute or two per side. Top with whipped cream, if you like.

MAKES 1 SERVING

NUTRITION PER SERVING (batter only)				
144 calories	0 g fat	6 g carbs	0 g fiber	26 g protein

BANANAS FOSTER
FRENCH TOAST

3 tablespoons (20 grams) vanilla or cinnamon protein powder

⅓ banana, heated and mashed

¼ cup liquid egg whites

½ teaspoon ground cinnamon

1 teaspoon maple syrup, plus more for drizzling

1 teaspoon imitation rum flavoring

1 large or 2 small, thick slices bread

2 tablespoons Vanilla Ice Cream (page 140), to top (optional)

1 Preheat a large pan over medium heat. Spray with a coat of cooking spray.

2 Mix the first six ingredients together in a wide bowl.

3 Soak the bread for a few minutes, making sure that there are no dry parts left, and place in the preheated pan.

4 Cook the French toast for a minute or two per side. Top with ice cream, if you like.

MAKES 1 SERVING

NUTRITION PER SERVING (batter only)				
170 calories	0 g fat	14 g carbs	1 g fiber	26 g protein

ZESTY ORANGE FRENCH TOAST

3 heaping tablespoons (20 grams) vanilla protein powder

¼ cup liquid egg whites

¼ cup orange juice

1 orange, zested

1 teaspoon honey

1 large or 2 small, thick slices bread

2 to 3 tablespoons light whipped cream, to top (optional)

1 Preheat a large pan over medium heat. Spray with a coat of cooking spray.

2 Mix the protein powder, egg whites, orange juice, orange zest, and honey together in a wide bowl.

3 Soak the bread for a few minutes, making sure that there are no dry parts left, and place in the preheated pan.

4 Cook the French toast for a minute or two per side. Top with whipped cream, if you like.

MAKES 1 SERVING

NUTRITION PER SERVING (batter only)				
162 calories	0 g fat	11 g carbs	0 g fiber	27 g protein

ESPRESSO FRENCH TOAST

3 heaping tablespoons (20 grams) chocolate protein powder

¼ cup liquid egg whites

1 tablespoon instant espresso powder

1 teaspoon cocoa powder

1 teaspoon agave syrup

1 large or 2 small, thick slices bread

2 to 3 tablespoons light whipped cream, to top (optional)

1 Preheat a large pan over medium heat. Spray with a coat of cooking spray.

2 Mix the protein powder, egg whites, espresso powder, cocoa powder, and agave syrup together in a wide bowl.

3 Soak the bread for a few minutes, making sure that there are no dry parts left, and place in the preheated pan.

4 Cook the French toast for a minute or two per side. Top with whipped cream, if you like.

MAKES 1 SERVING

NUTRITION PER SERVING (batter only)				
139 calories	0 g fat	5 g carbs	0 g fiber	26 g protein

BRIE AND PEAR FRENCH TOAST

3 heaping tablespoons (20 grams) vanilla or cinnamon protein powder

¼ cup liquid egg whites

1 teaspoon honey

1 large or 2 small, thick slices bread

½ ripe pear, sliced

1 tablespoon softened brie cheese, to top

1 Preheat a large pan over medium heat. Spray with a coat of cooking spray.

2 Mix the protein powder, egg whites, and honey together in a wide bowl.

3 Soak the bread for a few minutes, making sure that there are no dry parts left, and place in the preheated pan.

4 Cook the French toast for a minute or two per side and transfer to a plate.

5 Spray the pan again with cooking spray, and cook the pear slices for a minute or two per side.

6 Spread the brie on the finished French toast and top with the slices of pear.

MAKES 1 SERVING

NUTRITION PER SERVING (batter and toppings only)				
231 calories	4 g fat	18 g carbs	3 g fiber	29 g protein

WAFFLE FRENCH TOAST

2 squares waffles of choice
(pages 39 to 44)

¼ cup (30 grams) vanilla or other
protein powder

⅓ cup liquid egg whites

1 teaspoon agave syrup

1 teaspoon maple syrup, plus more
for drizzling

2 to 3 tablespoons light whipped
cream to top (optional)

1 Make waffles ahead of time.

2 Preheat a large pan over medium heat. Spray with a coat of cooking
spray.

3 Mix the protein powder, egg whites, and syrups together in a wide
bowl.

4 Soak the waffles for a few minutes, making sure that there are no dry
parts left, and place in the preheated pan.

5 Cook the waffle French toast for a minute or two per side. Top with
the maple syrup and whipped cream, if you like.

MAKES 1 SERVING

NUTRITION PER SERVING (batter only)				
133 calories	0 g fat	5 g carbs	0 g fiber	26 g protein

DOUGHNUTS AND SCONES

All of these doughnuts are baked, making them more cake-like than your usual fried doughnut, but one or two of them still feel like the ultimate breakfast treat! Even better, they won't leave you with a sugar crash an hour or two later. Frost them with any of the recipes on pages 166 to 175 for added protein and deliciousness!

CHOCOLATE CAKE DOUGHNUTS

1 cup flour

½ teaspoon baking soda

¼ teaspoon salt

½ cup (55 grams) chocolate protein powder

2 tablespoons cocoa powder

½ cup applesauce

⅓ cup Greek yogurt

¼ cup water or milk

3 tablespoons liquid egg whites

2 tablespoons oil

¼ cup sugar

¼ cup brown sugar

1 recipe Chocolate Avocado Frosting (page 166)

1 Preheat the oven to 350°F. Coat two doughnut pans with cooking spray.

2 Combine all ingredients in a large bowl and mix just until everything is incorporated. Portion the batter into doughnut pans. For regular-size doughnuts, bake 18 to 20 minutes, or for mini doughnuts, bake 12 minutes. Once the doughnuts are cooled, frost and serve, or refrigerate in a sealed container until serving.

MAKES 12 DOUGHNUTS

NUTRITION PER DOUGHNUT (without frosting)				
133 calories	0 g fat	5 g carbs	0 g fiber	26 g protein

APPLE CRUMBLE DOUGHNUTS

½ cup (55 grams) vanilla or cinnamon protein powder

1¼ cups flour

¼ cup oats

½ teaspoon baking soda

¼ teaspoon salt

3 tablespoons liquid egg whites

⅓ cup Greek yogurt

⅓ cup applesauce

½ cup brown sugar

1 Granny Smith apple, peeled and finely diced

¾ teaspoon ground cinnamon

1 teaspoon maple flavor or vanilla extract

FOR THE CRUMBLE TOPPING:

3 tablespoons (20 to 25 grams) vanilla protein powder

½ cup oats

½ teaspoon ground cinnamon

1 tablespoon applesauce

1 Preheat the oven to 350°F. Coat two doughnut pans with cooking spray.

2 Combine all of the doughnut ingredients in a large bowl and mix just until everything is incorporated. Portion the batter into doughnut pans.

3 In a small bowl, combine all of the crumble topping ingredients. Sprinkle evenly on all the doughnuts.

4 For regular-size doughnuts, bake for 18 to 20 minutes; for mini doughnuts, bake for 12 minutes.

MAKES 14 DOUGHNUTS

NUTRITION PER DOUGHNUT				
118 calories	3 g fat	18 g carbs	1 g fiber	7 g protein

PINEAPPLE UPSIDE-DOWN DOUGHNUTS

½ cup (55 grams) vanilla protein powder

½ cup applesauce

¼ cup Greek yogurt

2 tablespoons vegetable oil or coconut oil

½ cup liquid egg whites

⅓ cup sugar

1¾ cups flour

1 teaspoon baking soda

¼ teaspoon salt

1 (15-ounce) can pineapple chunks or rings in pineapple juice, drained

1 Preheat the oven to 350°F.

2 Coat two doughnut pans with cooking spray.

3 Combine all but the last ingredient in a large bowl and mix just until everything is incorporated.

4 Place the pineapple rings or chunks at the bottom of doughnut pans. Portion the batter into the doughnut pans.

5 For regular-size doughnuts, bake for 18 to 20 minutes; for mini doughnuts, bake for 12 minutes.

MAKES 15 DOUGHNUTS

NUTRITION PER DOUGHNUT				
115 calories	2 g fat	20 g carbs	2 g fiber	7 g protein

PUMPKIN DOUGHNUTS

½ cup (55 grams) vanilla or cinnamon protein powder

½ cup pumpkin puree

⅓ cup Greek yogurt

¼ cup milk

3 tablespoons liquid egg whites

½ cup sugar

1 teaspoon vanilla extract

1 cup flour

½ teaspoon baking soda

¼ teaspoon salt

1 teaspoon ground cinnamon

½ teaspoon ground ginger

½ teaspoon allspice

¼ teaspoon nutmeg

FOR THE FROSTING:

1 recipe Cream Cheese Frosting (page 169) or Pumpkin Cream Cheese Frosting (page 173)

1 Preheat the oven to 350°F. Coat two doughnut pans with cooking spray.

2 Combine all of the doughnut ingredients in a large bowl and mix just until everything is incorporated. Portion the batter into doughnut pans.

3 For regular-size doughnuts, bake for 18 to 20 minutes; for mini doughnuts, bake for 12 minutes.

4 Meanwhile, prepare frosting and refrigerate until using. Warm to room temperature before frosting the doughnuts.

5 Once the doughnuts are cooled, frost and serve, or refrigerate in a sealed container until ready to serve.

MAKES 12 DOUGHNUTS

NUTRITION PER DOUGHNUT (without frosting)				
124 calories	3 g fat	18 g carbs	2 g fiber	7 g protein

ARNOLD PALMER DOUGHNUTS

½ cup (55 grams) vanilla or lemon protein powder

½ cup applesauce

⅓ cup Greek yogurt

¼ cup milk

3 tablespoons liquid egg whites

½ cup sugar

2 tablespoons unsweetened instant tea powder

1 cup flour

½ teaspoon baking soda

¼ teaspoon salt

FOR THE FROSTING:

1 recipe Vanilla Silk Frosting (page 168)

1 teaspoons lemon extract

lemon zest, for finishing (optional)

1 Preheat the oven to 350°F. Coat two doughnut pans with cooking spray.

2 Combine all of the doughnut ingredients in a large bowl and mix just until everything is incorporated. Portion the batter into greased doughnut pans.

3 For regular-size doughnuts, bake for 18 to 20 minutes; for mini doughnuts, bake for 12 minutes.

4 Meanwhile, prepare frosting, adding in lemon extract and lemon zest, then refrigerate until using. Warm to room temperature before frosting the doughnuts.

5 Once the doughnuts are cooled, frost and serve or refrigerate in a sealed container until ready to serve.

MAKES 12 DOUGHNUTS

NUTRITION PER DOUGHNUT (without frosting)				
124 calories	3 g fat	18 g carbs	1 g fiber	7 g protein

S'MORES DOUGHNUTS

½ cup (55 grams) graham cracker, vanilla, chocolate protein powder

½ cup applesauce

⅓ cup Greek yogurt

¼ cup milk

3 tablespoons liquid egg whites

½ cup sugar

1 teaspoon vanilla extract

1 cup flour

½ teaspoon baking soda

¼ teaspoon salt

⅓ cup mini chocolate chips

⅓ cup mini marshmallows

FOR THE FROSTING:

1 recipe Chocolate Avocado Frosting (page 166) or Vanilla Silk Frosting (page 168)

2 graham crackers, crushed, to top

1 Preheat the oven to 350°F. Coat two doughnut pans with cooking spray.

2 Combine all of the ingredients except the frosting ingredients and the crushed graham crackers in a large bowl and mix just until everything is incorporated.

3 Portion the batter into doughnut pans.

4 For regular-size doughnuts, bake for 18 to 20 minutes; for mini doughnuts, bake for 12 minutes.

5 Meanwhile, prepare frosting and refrigerate until you're ready to use it. Warm to room temperature before frosting the doughnuts.

6 Once the doughnuts are cooled, frost and serve, or refrigerate in a sealed container until you're ready to serve them. Just before serving, top with crushed graham crackers.

MAKES 12 DOUGHNUTS

NUTRITION PER DOUGHNUT (without frosting)				
167 calories	5 g fat	25 g carbs	2 g fiber	8 g protein

FRENCH-TOASTED DOUGHNUTS

3 heaping tablespoons (20 grams) vanilla or other protein powder

¼ cup any milk or juice

¼ cup liquid egg whites

1 recipe doughnuts (pages 64–69)

Up to 3 tablespoons powdered sugar or stevia powder, for dusting

1 Follow the recipe instructions to make the doughnut of your choice.

2 Preheat a large pan over medium heat. Coat with cooking spray.

3 Combine the protein powder, milk or juice, and egg whites in a bowl.

4 Dip three premade doughnuts into the batter and allow each one to absorb as much of the liquid as possible on each side before moving it to the preheated pan.

5 Cook the doughnuts for a few minutes per side until browned. Remove to a plate and dust with the powdered sugar or stevia powder.

6 Serve immediately or refrigerate until ready to serve.

MAKES ENOUGH FOR 3 DOUGHNUTS

NUTRITION PER DOUGHNUT (batter only)				
70 calories	0 g fat	8 g carbs	0 g fiber	9 g protein

Tip: If there is any extra liquid, you can use it on more doughnuts or add enough ground flaxseed to make pancakes, and cook the batter in the pan.

VANILLA SCONES

Once you start making these scones, you won't want to stop! The way that the butter (or coconut oil) is combined with the dry ingredients is a biscuit technique that creates a uniquely soft, fluffy texture, even using 100 percent whole wheat flour. With all the protein and fiber in each one of these mini scones, you can enjoy a few and call it a balanced breakfast!

⅔ cup (80 grams) vanilla protein powder

3 cups flour

3 tablespoons sugar

2½ teaspoons baking powder

½ teaspoon baking soda

½ teaspoon salt

8 tablespoons butter or coconut oil

⅓ cup Greek yogurt

1 cup milk

1 teaspoon vanilla extract

1 egg

1½ teaspoons vanilla bean paste (optional)

3 tablespoons liquid egg whites

1 tablespoon coarse sugar

1 Preheat the oven to 425°F. Spray two or three baking sheets with cooking spray.

2 Combine the first six ingredients in a bowl or food processor.

3 Chop the butter into tiny pieces and sprinkle them into the flour mixture, or drop the coconut oil in by the spoonful. Using the food processor or a pastry blender, combine the flour and butter/coconut oil until no clumps remain.

4 Combine the mixture with the yogurt, milk, vanilla, and egg in a bowl with a spatula. You may need to use a stand mixer or your hands to fully combine all the ingredients, as it will be a somewhat dry dough.

5 Once the dough comes together, cut it into four equal pieces and place one section on a dry, clean surface. Flatten the dough, spread on one-fourth of the vanilla bean paste (if using), and fold it over itself.

6 Press down, and repeat a few more times. Shape the dough into a square about ½-inch thick. Cut the square in half, and then use a knife to cut each rectangle into alternating triangles. Repeat the process with the remaining sections.

7 Place the triangles on the prepared baking sheet, with some space around them. Brush the rolls with the egg whites and sprinkle with the sugar. Bake for 12 to 14 minutes or until cooked through but still soft.

MAKES 25 SCONES

NUTRITION PER SCONE				
108 calories	4 g fat	12 g carbs	2 g fiber	5 g protein

JAVA SCONES

2 tablespoons instant espresso or coffee powder

¼ cup chocolate covered espresso beans (optional)

Follow the instructions for the Vanilla Scones, substituting the above ingredient(s) for the vanilla bean paste.

MAKES 25 SCONES

NUTRITION PER SCONE				
108 calories	4 g fat	12 g carbs	2 g fiber	5 g protein

CINNAMON RAISIN SCONES

1 cup raisins

2 teaspoons ground cinnamon

Follow the instructions for the Vanilla Scones, substituting the above ingredient(s) for the vanilla bean paste.

MAKES 25 SCONES

NUTRITION PER SCONE				
138 calories	4 g fat	15 g carbs	3 g fiber	5 g protein

NUTELLA SCONES

¼ cup Nutella (or other hazelnut-chocolate spread)

Follow the instructions for the Vanilla Scones, substituting the above ingredient(s) for the vanilla bean paste.

MAKES 25 SCONES

NUTRITION PER SCONE				
138 calories	5 g fat	14 g carbs	2 g fiber	5 g protein

GINGER LIME SCONES

1 teaspoon lime or lemon extract

2 tablespoons freshly grated ginger

2 limes, zested

Follow the instructions for the Vanilla Scones, substituting the above ingredient(s) for the vanilla bean paste.

MAKES 25 SCONES

NUTRITION PER SCONE				
108 calories	4 g fat	12 g carbs	2 g fiber	5 g protein

STRAWBERRY VANILLA SCONES

Try using strawberry-flavored protein powder in this recipe!

½ cup chopped fresh strawberries

3 tablespoons honey or agave syrup

Follow the instructions for the Vanilla Scones, substituting the above ingredient(s) for the vanilla bean paste.

MAKES 25 SCONES

NUTRITION PER SCONE				
111 calories	4 g fat	13 g carbs	3 g fiber	5 g protein

BLUEBERRY LEMON SCONES

1 lemon, zested

½ cup fresh or frozen blueberries

Follow the instructions for the Vanilla Scones, substituting the above ingredient(s) for the vanilla bean paste.

MAKES 25 SCONES

NUTRITION PER SCONE				
116 calories	4 g fat	13 g carbs	3 g fiber	5 g protein

MATCHA PISTACHIO SCONES

3 tablespoons finely crushed pistachios

¼ cup matcha green tea powder

Follow the instructions for the Vanilla Scones, substituting the above ingredient(s) for the vanilla bean paste.

MAKES 25 SCONES

NUTRITION PER SCONE				
118 calories	5 g fat	13 g carbs	2 g fiber	6 g protein

CHOCOLATE SCONES

⅔ cup (80 grams) chocolate protein powder

3 cups flour

¼ cup cocoa powder

3 tablespoons brown sugar

2½ teaspoons baking powder

½ teaspoon baking soda

½ teaspoon salt

8 tablespoons butter or coconut oil

⅓ cup Greek yogurt

1 cup milk

1 egg

1 teaspoon vanilla extract

3 tablespoons liquid egg whites

1 tablespoon coarse sugar

1 Preheat the oven to 425°F. Spray two or three baking sheets with cooking spray.

2 Combine the first seven ingredients in a bowl or food processor. Chop the butter into tiny pieces and sprinkle them into the flour mixture, or drop the coconut oil in by the spoonful. Using a food processor or a pastry blender, combine the flour and butter/coconut oil until no clumps remain.

3 Combine the mixture with the yogurt, milk, egg, and vanilla in a bowl with a spatula. You may need to use a stand mixer or your hands to fully combine all the ingredients, as it will be a somewhat dry dough.

4 Once the dough comes together, cut it into four equal pieces and place one section on a dry, clean surface. Flatten the dough, and fold it over itself.

5 Press down, and repeat a few more times. Shape the dough into a square about ½-inch thick. Cut the square in half, and then use a knife to cut each rectangle into alternating triangles. Repeat the process with the remaining sections.

6 Place the triangles on the prepared baking sheet with some space around them. Brush the rolls with the egg whites and sprinkle with the sugar. Bake for 12 to 14 minutes or until cooked through but still soft.

MAKES 25 SCONES

NUTRITION PER SCONE				
108 calories	4 g fat	12 g carbs	2 g fiber	5 g protein

CHOCOLATE BLACKBERRY SCONES

¾ cup chopped fresh blackberries

1 Follow the instructions for the Chocolate Scones, adding in the above ingredient(s) right after flattening out the dough.

2 Incorporate the added ingredient(s) as you would in any of the Vanilla Scone variations.

3 Complete the remaining steps to finish the scones.

MAKES 25 SCONES

NUTRITION PER SCONE				
114 calories	4 g fat	13 g carbs	3 g fiber	5 g protein

TRIPLE CHOCOLATE SCONES

½ cup chocolate spread (such as Nutella)

⅓ cup mini chocolate chips

1 Follow the instructions for the Chocolate Scones, adding in the above ingredient(s) right after flattening out the dough.

2 Incorporate the added ingredient(s) as you would in any of the Vanilla Scone variations.

3 Complete the remaining steps to finish the scones.

MAKES 25 SCONES

NUTRITION PER SCONE				
140 calories	6 g fat	15 g carbs	2 g fiber	5 g protein

CHOCOLATE PEANUT BUTTER SCONES

½ cup peanut butter

¼ cup (30 grams) vanilla or chocolate protein powder

1 In a small bowl, combine the peanut butter with the protein powder and set aside before making the scones.

2 Follow the instructions for the Chocolate Scones, adding in the above ingredient(s) right after flattening out the dough.

3 Incorporate the added ingredient(s) as you would in any of the Vanilla Scone variations.

4 Complete the remaining steps to finish the scones.

MAKES 25 SCONES

NUTRITION PER SCONE				
142 calories	7 g fat	13 g carbs	2 g fiber	7 g protein

MUFFINS AND QUICK BREADS

I do love a good slice of banana bread or some soft muffins, but I really love it if I also know it's good for me! If you bake a batch over the weekend, you can have some for your Sunday brunch and refrigerate the rest for a quick breakfast or snack throughout the week.

MONKEY MOCHA COFFEE CAKE

If you're trying to reduce your carb intake or just increase your protein intake, these fluffy muffins can be a big help. With absolutely no flour, they are surprisingly great substitutes for your usual morning muffin.

½ cup (55 grams) chocolate protein powder

2 very ripe bananas

⅔ cup brewed coffee

¼ cup coconut oil

½ cup brown sugar

2¼ cups flour

1 cup oat flour

½ teaspoon salt

1½ teaspoons baking powder

½ teaspoon baking soda

FOR THE CRUMBLY TOPPING (OPTIONAL):

2 tablespoons chopped dates

2 tablespoons chocolate-covered espresso beans

2 tablespoons rolled oats

1 tablespoon brewed coffee or water

1 Preheat the oven to 350°F. Coat a 9 x 9-inch square cake pan with cooking spray.

2 Blend together the first five ingredients until very smooth.

3 Whisk together flour, oat flour, salt, baking powder, and baking soda in a medium bowl. Pour in the banana mixture and stir just until combined. Pour the batter into the prepared cake pan.

4 In a food processor, process the crumbly topping ingredients together, if using. Sprinkle it across the top of the cake batter.

5 Bake in the oven for 35 to 40 minutes or until a toothpick inserted in the center comes out clean.

MAKES 12 SERVINGS

NUTRITION PER SERVING				
260 calories	7 g fat	41 g carbs	5 g fiber	9 g protein

SNICKERDOODLE MUFFINS

½ cup (55 grams) vanilla or cinnamon protein powder

¾ cup liquid egg whites

1 tablespoon coconut oil, melted

1 tablespoon Greek yogurt

3 tablespoons ground flaxseed

½ teaspoon ground cinnamon

½ teaspoon baking powder

⅛ teaspoon salt

FOR THE TOPPING:

3 tablespoons sugar

1 tablespoon ground cinnamon

1 Preheat the oven to 400°F. Coat a 12-cup muffin tin with baking spray.

2 Combine all ingredients through salt in a medium bowl. Portion the batter out evenly between eight of the muffin cups.

3 To make the topping, combine the sugar and cinnamon in a small bowl. Sift evenly on top of all the muffins.

4 Bake for about 9 minutes or just until the muffins look/feel fluffy. Allow to cool for a few minutes before removing gently from the muffin tray.

MAKES 8 MUFFINS | LOW-CARB | GLUTEN-FREE

NUTRITION PER SERVING				
100 calories	5 g fat	3 g carbs	2 g fiber	11 g protein

BLUEBERRY MUFFINS

½ cup (55 grams) vanilla protein powder

¾ cup liquid egg whites

1 tablespoon coconut oil, melted

1 tablespoon Greek yogurt

3 tablespoons ground flaxseed

½ teaspoon baking powder

⅛ teaspoon salt

⅓ cup fresh or frozen blueberries, reserved

3 tablespoons crushed walnuts, pecans, or almonds (optional)

1 Preheat the oven to 400°F.

2 Coat a 12-cup muffin tin with baking spray.

3 Combine all ingredients through salt in a medium bowl. Gently mix in the blueberries.

4 Portion the batter out evenly between eight of the muffin cups and sprinkle the crushed nuts onto each muffin.

5 Bake for about 9 minutes or just until the muffins look/feel fluffy. Allow to cool for a few minutes before removing gently from the muffin tray.

MAKES 8 MUFFINS | LOW-CARB | GLUTEN-FREE

NUTRITION PER SERVING				
109 calories	5 g fat	4 g carbs	3 g fiber	11 g protein

CHOCOLATE MUFFIN TOPS

½ cup (55 grams) chocolate protein powder

¾ cup liquid egg whites

1 tablespoon coconut oil, melted

3 tablespoons ground flaxseed

½ teaspoon baking powder

⅛ teaspoon salt

1 Preheat the oven to 400°F.

2 Coat a 12-cup muffin tin with baking spray.

3 Combine all of the ingredients in a medium bowl. Portion the batter out evenly between eight of the muffin cups.

4 Bake for about 9 minutes or just until the muffins look/feel fluffy. Allow to cool for a few minutes before removing gently from the muffin tray.

MAKES 8 MUFFINS | LOW-CARB | GLUTEN-FREE

NUTRITION PER MUFFIN				
100 calories	5 g fat	3 g carbs	2 g fiber	11 g protein

CHOCOLATE BANANA NUT BREAD

Let's face it—everything is better with chocolate. If there is one thing better than banana bread, it's chocolate banana bread. The nuts add a nice crunch and extra nutrition!

⅔ cup (80 grams) chocolate protein powder

2 large very ripe bananas

½ cup coconut oil, melted

½ cup Greek yogurt

⅔ cup sugar

⅔ cup stevia

2 eggs

1 teaspoon vanilla extract

4 tablespoons cocoa powder

2½ cups flour

⅔ cup oat flour

⅓ cup chopped walnuts or pecans

2 teaspoons baking powder

1 teaspoon baking soda

½ teaspoon salt

1 Preheat the oven to 350°F.

2 In a stand mixer fitted with the whisk attachment or in a food processor, combine the first eight ingredients. Mix in the remaining ingredients. Scoop the batter into two greased 8 x 4-inch loaf pans and bake for 45 to 50 minutes or until just done.

3 Allow to cool for at least 10 minutes in the pans before running a knife around the edges and removing, or leave in the pan and store, covered, at room temperature for up to 2 days. Alternatively, freeze in a freezer-safe bag or store in a sealed container in the refrigerator for up to a week.

MAKES 12 SLICES

NUTRITION PER SLICE				
313 calories	13 g fat	40 g carbs	4 g fiber	12 g protein

MINI BANANA LOAVES

Slices of these dense, moist banana loaves make energizing breakfasts or snacks and can be made gluten-free just by using gluten-free certified oats.

½ cup (55 grams) vanilla or cinnamon protein powder

2 medium, very ripe bananas

½ cup liquid egg whites

2 tablespoons ground flaxseed

3 tablespoons agave syrup

1 cup quick oats or oat flour

⅓ cup coconut flour

¾ teaspoon cinnamon

¼ teaspoon salt

1½ teaspoons baking powder

1 Preheat the oven to 350°F.

2 In a stand mixer fitted with the whisk attachment or in a food processor, combine the first five ingredients. Mix in the remaining ingredients.

3 Scoop the batter into two small greased 7 x 3-inch loaf pans and bake for 35 to 40 minutes or until just done.

4 Allow to cool at least 10 minutes in the pans before running a knife around the edges and removing, or leave in the pan and store, covered, at room temperature for up to 2 days. Alternatively, freeze in a freezer-safe bag or store in a sealed container in the refrigerator for up to a week.

MAKES 10 SLICES | GLUTEN-FREE

NUTRITION PER SLICE				
125 calories	2 g fat	20 g carbs	3 g fiber	8 g protein

CHERRY BEET MUFFINS

Muffins made with both cherries and beets are like superheroes for your heart. If you like all the nutrition in these but want less sugar in your life, feel free to swap out the sugar with stevia or erythritol.

½ (15-ounce) can or 1 cup pitted cherries

½ (15-ounce) can or 1 cup cooked beets, drained

⅔ cup (80 grams) vanilla protein powder

3 tablespoons liquid egg whites

1 cup sugar

1½ cups flour

1 teaspoon baking soda

½ teaspoon salt

1 Preheat the oven to 350°F. Coat a 12-cup muffin tin with baking spray.

2 Strain the cherries from the packing water over a bowl. Measure out 1 cup of the drained cherries and ¼ cup of the water it was in and transfer to a food processor.

3 Add the beets, protein powder, egg whites, and sugar to the food processor and puree. Add the remaining ingredients and mix well until just combined. Portion the batter out evenly into the muffin cups.

4 Bake for 18 to 20 minutes or until just baked through, being careful not to overbake. Remove from the muffin pan and allow to cool completely on a wire rack.

MAKES 12 MUFFINS

NUTRITION PER MUFFIN				
163 calories	0 g fat	29 g carbs	2 g fiber	8 g protein

STRAWBERRY COCONUT COFFEE CAKE

Extremely moist and fluffy, this is a favorite coffee cake of mine. It also looks pretty impressive, so I love making this one for guests when I can.

⅓ cup (40 grams) vanilla or strawberry protein powder

2 cups flour

1 teaspoon baking soda

½ teaspoon baking powder

½ teaspoon salt

½ cup coconut oil

⅔ cup Greek yogurt

¾ cup sugar

1½ teaspoons vanilla extract

1 cup finely chopped strawberries

⅓ cup sweetened coconut shreds, to top

1 Preheat the oven to 350°F. Coat an 8 x 8-inch pan with cooking spray.

2 Mix all of the ingredients except for the coconut shreds together in a bowl. Pour the batter into the pan and spread out evenly.

3 Sprinkle the coconut shreds on top of the batter.

4 Bake for about 30 minutes or until just baked through in the center. Remove to a cooling rack and cool to room temperature before slicing.

MAKES 12 SERVINGS

NUTRITION PER SERVING				
237 calories	11 g fat	31 g carbs	3 g fiber	6 g protein

FIG WALNUT COFFEE CAKE

The fig walnut crumble on the coffee cake is simply out of this world. I can't get around how tasty it is on the soft vanilla coffee cake.

1¼ cups flour

⅔ cup (80 grams) vanilla protein powder

¾ teaspoon baking soda

¼ teaspoon salt

½ cup sugar

½ cup Greek yogurt

½ cup applesauce

2 tablespoons oil

FOR THE FIG CRUMBLE:

1 cup dried figs

2 tablespoons lemon juice

¼ cup sugar

¼ cup walnuts

1 Preheat the oven to 350°F. Coat an 8 x 8-inch pan with cooking spray.

2 Mix all of the ingredients for the coffee cake together in a bowl. Pour the batter into the pan and spread out evenly.

3 In a food processor, pulse all of the fig crumble ingredients together to make a coarse crumble. Sprinkle the fig crumble across the top of the batter and use a knife to slightly swirl the crumble into the top of the batter.

4 Bake for about 30 minutes or until just baked through in the center. Remove to a cooling rack and cool to room temperature before slicing.

MAKES 12 SERVINGS

NUTRITION PER SERVING				
221 calories	4 g fat	40 g carbs	3 g fiber	8 g protein

ESPRESSO BREAKFAST BARS

I'm of the opinion that there is no such thing as coffee-flavor overload and will happily pair an espresso-flavored breakfast bar with my morning Joe. That's not just me, right?

¼ cup (30 grams) vanilla, chocolate, or coffee protein powder

1 cup oats

1 cup flour

¾ teaspoon baking soda

¼ teaspoon salt

⅓ cup liquid egg whites

½ cup applesauce

½ cup sugar

⅓ cup chopped walnuts

2 tablespoons espresso powder

1 Preheat the oven to 350°F. Coat an 8 x 8-inch pan with cooking spray.

2 Mix all of the ingredients together in a bowl. Pour the mixture into the pan and spread out evenly.

3 Bake for 20 to 25 minutes or until just baked through in the center. Remove to a cooling rack and cool to room temperature before cutting into bars.

MAKES 12 SERVINGS

NUTRITION PER SERVING				
131 calories	4 g fat	22 g carbs	3 g fiber	6 g protein

BERRY COFFEE CAKE

Oh, berry coffee cake. You do make my heart skip a beat! All those delicious berries always keep me coming back for more.

heaping ½ cup (70 grams) vanilla protein powder

¼ cup oil

¼ cup applesauce

½ cup Greek yogurt

2 eggs

½ cup sugar

1 teaspoon vanilla extract *or* 1 tablespoon lime juice

1¼ cups flour

1 teaspoon baking powder

½ teaspoon salt

½ cup fresh raspberries

½ cup fresh blackberries

1 Preheat the oven to 350°F. Coat a 9 x 5-inch loaf pan with cooking spray.

2 Combine the first seven ingredients together in a bowl or mixer. Whisk in the flour, baking powder, and salt, and add them to the wet mixture. Mix to combine.

3 Gently fold in the raspberries and blackberries. Pour the batter into the cake pan and spread out evenly.

4 Bake for 45 to 55 minutes or until just baked through in the center. Remove to a cooling rack and cool to room temperature before slicing.

MAKES 12 SERVINGS

NUTRITION PER SERVING				
152 calories	3 g fat	19 g carbs	2 g fiber	8 g protein

BANANA OAT MUFFINS

If you couldn't tell, I'm a bit of a junkie for baking with banana. For one thing, bananas are delicious. For another, they're full of potassium and good carbs that help sweeten your treats that help you recover from your workouts. Also, it's just the thing to do with a past-its-prime banana!

½ cup (55 grams) vanilla, banana, or cinnamon protein powder

1 large very ripe banana

1 egg

¼ cup liquid egg whites

¼ cup oil

¼ cup applesauce

½ teaspoon maple flavor *or* 1 teaspoon vanilla extract

¼ cup maple syrup

1⅓ cups flour

1 cup oats

¼ teaspoon salt

¼ teaspoon baking soda

FOR THE CRUMBLE TOPPING:

½ cup pecans

3 tablespoons (20 grams) vanilla protein powder

¼ cup oats

2 tablespoons applesauce

1 Preheat the oven to 350°F. Coat a 12-cup muffin tin with baking spray.

2 Combine the first eight ingredients in a stand mixer or in a food processor. Add the flour, oats, salt, and baking soda to the batter and mix well until just combined. Portion the batter out evenly into the muffin cups.

3 In a food processor, pulse the topping ingredients until they resemble a coarse meal. Evenly distribute the crumble on top of the muffin batter.

4 Bake for about 18 minutes or until just baked through, being careful not to overbake. Remove from the muffin pan and allow to cool completely on a wire rack.

MAKES 12 MUFFINS

NUTRITION PER MUFFIN				
210 calories	9 g fat	24 g carbs	10 g fiber	3 g protein

OATMEAL MUFFINS

It's like an oatmeal cookie… but in muffin form!

½ cup (55 grams) vanilla or cinnamon protein powder

6 tablespoons Greek yogurt

¼ cup applesauce

¼ cup brown sugar

¼ cup stevia

¼ cup butter, melted

2 tablespoons ground flaxseed

1 teaspoon ground cinnamon

½ teaspoon ground ginger

¾ cup rolled oats

½ cup flour

⅛ teaspoon salt

1. Preheat the oven to 350°F. Coat a 12-cup muffin tin with baking spray.

2. Combine the first 9 ingredients in a large bowl. Add the remaining ingredients and mix well until just combined. Portion the batter out evenly into the muffin cups.

3. Bake for 16 to 17 minutes or until just baked through, being careful not to overbake. Remove from the muffin pan and allow to cool completely on a wire rack.

MAKES 12 MUFFINS

NUTRITION PER MUFFIN				
154 calories	9 g fat	14 g carbs	2 g fiber	7 g protein

CHOCOLATE PEANUT BUTTER BANANA MUFFINS

Some of the best things come in one muffin! I highly recommend picking up a container of PB2 powdered peanut butter as it can come in handy whenever you want a little extra peanut flavor without the extra fat and calories. If you don't have it, try substituting it with 2 tablespoons of peanut butter–flavored protein powder.

½ cup (55 grams) peanut butter protein powder

4 large, very ripe bananas

⅓ cup coconut oil, melted

½ cup stevia

½ cup brown sugar

1 egg

2 tablespoons PB2

1 cup flour

¼ cup ground flaxseed

¼ cup cocoa powder

1½ teaspoons baking powder

½ teaspoon salt

1 Preheat the oven to 350°F. Coat a 12-cup muffin tin with baking spray.

2 Combine the first six ingredients in a stand mixer or a food processor. Add the remaining ingredients and mix well until just combined. Portion the batter out evenly into the muffin cups.

3 Bake for 18 to 20 minutes or until just baked through, being careful not to overbake. Remove from the muffin pan and allow to cool completely on a wire rack.

MAKES 12 MUFFINS

NUTRITION PER MUFFIN				
208 calories	8 g fat	28 g carbs	4 g fiber	7 g protein

CORNBREAD MUFFINS

Cornbread is a must-have on so many occasions, so it's never a bad idea to have a protein-packed, healthier version on hand for when you don't want to make any health or taste sacrifices!

½ cup (55 grams) vanilla protein powder

1½ cups yellow cornmeal

1 cup flour

1½ teaspoons baking powder

½ teaspoon salt

1 cup milk

⅔ cup applesauce

⅓ cup coconut oil, melted

¼ cup brown sugar

2 eggs

1 Preheat the oven to 350°F. Coat a 12-cup muffin tin with baking spray.

2 Combine the first five ingredients in a large bowl. Add the remaining ingredients and mix well until just combined. Portion the batter out evenly into greased muffin cups.

3 Bake for about 16 minutes or until just baked through, being careful not to overbake. Remove from the muffin pan and allow to cool completely on a wire rack.

MAKES 12 SERVINGS

NUTRITION PER SERVING				
198 calories	8 g fat	25 g carbs	3 g fiber	8 g protein

PEAR ALMOND COFFEE CAKE

There's just something about the combination of pear and almond flavors that works so well. Put together in a dense coffee cake, it's the best!

6 tablespoons Greek yogurt	½ cup flour
6 tablespoons applesauce	1 teaspoon baking powder
⅓ cup brown sugar	⅛ teaspoon salt
⅓ cup stevia	½ pear, finely chopped
¼ cup liquid egg whites	½ pear, thinly sliced
¼ teaspoon almond extract	¼ cup sliced almonds
⅓ cup (40 grams) vanilla protein powder	2 tablespoons brown sugar

1 Preheat the oven to 350°F. Coat a 9 x 5-inch loaf pan with cooking spray.

2 Mix the first eleven ingredients together in a bowl. Pour the batter into the cake pan and spread it out evenly.

3 Lay the sliced pear on the top of the coffee cake batter and sprinkle the sliced almonds and brown sugar on top.

4 Bake for about 40 minutes or until just baked through in the center. Remove to a cooling rack and cool to room temperature before slicing.

MAKES 10 SERVINGS

NUTRITION PER SERVING				
110 calories	2 g fat	16 g carbs	2 g fiber	7 g protein

PEACHES AND CREAM COFFEE CAKE

Believe me when I say you're gonna want to try this one! It's like having a cheesecake combined with your coffee cake and makes the best treat whenever peaches are available!

⅓ cup (40 grams), plus 2½ tablespoons (16 grams) vanilla protein powder, divided

½ cup applesauce

¼ cup coconut oil

⅓ cup sugar

3 ounces reduced-fat cream cheese

½ cup rolled oats

½ cup flour

1 teaspoon baking powder

¼ teaspoon salt

1 large, pitted peach

2 ounces cream cheese

1 Preheat the oven to 350°F. Coat an 8 x 8-inch cake pan with cooking spray.

2 Mix the ⅓ cup of protein powder, along with the next eight ingredients together in a bowl. Puree the peach and mix half the puree into the cake batter. Pour the batter into the cake pan and spread it out evenly.

3 Blend the remaining peach puree with the cream cheese and remaining protein powder. Swirl the cream cheese mixture into the top of the coffee cake batter.

4 Bake for 25 to 30 minutes, or until just baked through in the center. Remove to a cooling rack and cool to room temperature before slicing.

MAKES 12 SERVINGS

NUTRITION PER SERVING				
158 calories	8 g fat	15 g carbs	1 g fiber	7 g protein

SAVORY RECIPES

Plain protein powder can be used to ramp up the nutritional value of almost anything you can think of, from sauces to soups to pizzas! These recipes can help make vegetarian and vegan meals more satisfying and energizing and make any meal healthier by replacing traditional ingredients (like cream or flour) with protein powder.

BAKED BUTTERY DUMPLINGS

These little dumplings are dense and buttery—perfect for popping into a stew or eaten like biscuits. The best thing is you can enjoy them even on a low-carb diet!

⅔ cup (80 grams) plain protein powder

⅓ cup coconut flour

2 tablespoons ground flaxseed

1½ teaspoons baking soda

¼ teaspoon cream of tartar

¼ cup cold butter, chopped

2 tablespoons oil

2 eggs

½ teaspoon salt

1 tablespoon agave nectar or honey

6 tablespoons water

1 Preheat the oven to 350°F.

2 Blend the first six ingredients together in a food processor or using a pastry blender until the butter is distributed uniformly.

3 Heat the oil in a large pan over medium-high heat.

4 Add the remaining ingredients to the blender and combine to make a thick dough. Roll into 1½-inch-thick dumplings and place into the preheated pan.

5 Cook dumplings on all sides until browned and transfer to a baking sheet. Bake for 15 minutes or until cooked through.

MAKES 15 DUMPLINGS | LOW-CARB | GLUTEN-FREE

NUTRITION PER DUMPLING				
89 calories	6 g fat	3 g carbs	1 g fiber	5 g protein

PIZZA CRUST

I love having a low-carb option for one of my favorite foods—and it isn't just a tortilla-crust pizza! This crust really puffs up similar to a thick, doughy pizza, which can be really nice when trying to stick to a low-carb diet. Use any sauce, grated cheese, and toppings you like to make this pizza delicious!

⅓ cup (40 grams) plain protein powder

2 tablespoons ground flaxseed

1 teaspoon olive oil

½ teaspoon garlic powder

⅛ teaspoon salt

½ cup liquid egg whites

2 to 4 tablespoons each of sauce, grated cheese, and toppings

1 Heat a medium nonstick frying pan coated with cooking spray over medium heat.

2 In a medium bowl, mix all of the ingredients together well. Form the dough into a ball and press into a flat circle about ½-inch thick on a clean surface. Move to the heated pan and cook until the bottom is crisped and lightly browned. Flip and cook the other side just until done. Transfer to a baking sheet.

3 Top the pizza dough with sauce, cheese, and your favorite toppings. Place under the broiler to cook for about 2 minutes. DO NOT walk away! The broiler can easily burn the pizza. Remove from the oven and cut into slices.

MAKES 1 PIZZA | LOW-CARB | GLUTEN-FREE

NUTRITION FOR 1 PIZZA CRUST (Without toppings)				
323 calories	11 g fat	5 g carbs	4 g fiber	50 g protein

CHEESY BUNS

Believe it or not, you don't actually need flour to make a soft, fluffy muffin. These Cheesy Buns are really tasty alongside soup or cut in half and made into a mini cheese or ham sandwich!

¾ cup (90 grams) plain protein powder

¼ cup ground flaxseed

¾ teaspoon baking powder

1 cup liquid egg whites

1 tablespoon coconut oil, melted

½ cup any shredded cheese

chopped onions or chives

½ teaspoon onion powder

½ teaspoon garlic powder

½ teaspoon salt

pinch of salt, to top

1 Preheat the oven to 400°F.

2 Mix all of the ingredients together in a bowl.

3 Coat a muffin pan with baking spray. Portion the batter out evenly between eight of the muffin cups.

4 Bake for about 12 minutes, or just until the buns start to brown on the sides and look/feel fluffy. Allow to cool a few minutes before removing gently from the muffin tray.

MAKES 8 BUNS | LOW-CARB | GLUTEN-FREE

NUTRITION PER BUN				
105 calories	5 g fat	1 g carbs	1 g fiber	13 g protein

BEST CAULIFLOWER MASHED "POTATOES"

This recipe tastes so much like regular mashed potatoes, you'll never need the real traditional kind again. And, with all this protein, it's a great addition to a vegetarian meal!

1 head cauliflower, roughly chopped

½ cup (55 grams) plain protein powder

¼ cup butter

¾ teaspoon garlic powder

½ teaspoon onion powder

½ teaspoon ground white pepper

½ teaspoon salt

1 Preheat the oven to 400°F.

2 Roast the chopped cauliflower on a pan in the center of the oven until soft, about 25 minutes.

3 In a blender, puree the roasted cauliflower together with the remaining ingredients.

4 Add seasonings, to taste.

MAKES 10 SERVINGS | LOW-CARB | GLUTEN-FREE

NUTRITION PER SERVING				
126 calories	5 g fat	5 g carbs	2 g fiber	17 g protein

GNOCCHI

Gnocchi is always a deliciously hearty base for a pasta dish, but I love that this version has drastically lower carbs and a ton of protein, allowing me to fit pasta into any meal plan. Toss the finished gnocchi with sauce or even add it to a soup.

¾ cup (90 grams) plain protein powder

⅓ cup (40 grams) garbanzo bean flour

¼ cup liquid egg whites

1 egg

1 tablespoon olive oil

½ teaspoon garlic

½ teaspoon salt

1 Blend all of the ingredients together in a food processor until it forms a ball of dough. Scoop out teaspoon-sized portions and roll into balls.

2 Meanwhile, bring a pot of well-salted water to a boil. Once the water is boiling, drop all the gnocchi into the water.

3 Boil for 4 to 5 minutes, and then drain in a large colander.

4 Serve with any pasta sauce.

MAKES 4 SERVINGS | LOW-CARB | GLUTEN-FREE

NUTRITION PER SERVING				
175 calories	5 g fat	6 g carbs	2 g fiber	25 g protein

FLUFFY DINNER ROLLS

These rolls are definitely some of the best I've ever made or eaten! They come out light and fluffy every time, with a perfectly buttery flavor. Make them anytime—they go with everything!

⅔ cup (80 grams) plain protein powder

3 cups flour

3 tablespoons sugar

2½ teaspoons baking powder

½ teaspoon baking soda

½ teaspoon salt

8 tablespoons butter or coconut oil

⅓ cup Greek yogurt

1 cup milk

1 egg

3 tablespoons liquid egg whites

1 teaspoon coarse salt

1 Preheat the oven to 425°F. Spray two or three baking sheets with cooking spray.

2 Combine the first six ingredients in a bowl or food processor.

3 Chop the butter into tiny pieces and sprinkle them into the flour mixture, or drop the coconut oil in by the spoonful. Using the food processor or a pastry blender, combine the flour and butter/coconut oil until no more clumps remain.

4 In a large bowl, combine the flour mixture and the yogurt, milk, and egg with a spatula. You may need to use a stand mixer or your hands to fully combine all the ingredients, as it will be a somewhat dry dough.

5 Once the dough comes together, cut it into four equal pieces and place one section on a dry, clean surface. Flatten the dough, and fold it over itself. Press down, and repeat a few more times. Shape the dough into a square about ½-inch thick.

6 Cut the square in half, and then use a knife to cut each rectangle into alternating triangles. Repeat the process with the remaining sections.

7 Place the triangles on the prepared baking sheet with some space around them, and brush the rolls with the liquid egg whites and sprinkle with the salt. Bake 12 to 14 minutes, or until cooked through but still soft.

MAKES 25 ROLLS

NUTRITION PER ROLL				
108 calories	4 g fat	12 g carbs	2 g fiber	5 g protein

GARLIC BREAD BUNS

When you want garlic bread, this will be your new go-to recipe! It's a perfect accompaniment for any pasta dish or soup.

⅔ cup (80 grams) plain protein powder

3 cups flour

3 tablespoons sugar

2½ teaspoons baking powder

½ teaspoon baking soda

½ teaspoon salt

8 tablespoons butter or coconut oil

⅓ cup Greek yogurt

1 cup milk

1 egg

4 large cloves garlic, minced

¼ cup fresh basil leaves, chopped

3 tablespoons liquid egg whites

2 teaspoons garlic powder

1 teaspoon coarse salt

1 Preheat the oven to 425°F. Spray two or three baking sheets with cooking spray.

2 Combine the first six ingredients in a bowl or food processor. Chop the butter into tiny pieces and sprinkle them into the flour mixture, or drop the coconut oil in by the spoonful. Using the food processor or a pastry blender, combine the flour and butter/coconut oil until no more clumps remain.

3 In a large bowl, combine the flour mixture and the mixture with the yogurt, milk, and egg in a bowl with a spatula. You may need to use a stand mixer or your hands to fully combine all the ingredients, as it will be a somewhat dry dough.

4 Once the dough comes together, cut it into four equal pieces and place one section on a dry, clean surface. Flatten the dough, sprinkle it with one-fourth of the minced garlic and basil, and fold it over itself.

5 Press down, and repeat a few more times. Shape the dough into a square about ½-inch thick. Cut the square in half, and then use a knife to cut each rectangle into alternating triangles. Repeat the process with the remaining sections.

6 Place the triangles on the prepared baking sheet, with some space around them. Brush the rolls with the egg whites and sprinkle with the salt and garlic powder. Bake 12 to 14 minutes, or until cooked through but still soft.

MAKES 25 BUNS

NUTRITION PER BUN				
108 calories	4 g fat	12 g carbs	2 g fiber	5 g protein

BACON AND SHALLOT ROLLS

Not being the hugest bacon aficionado, I was surprised to find that these are actually my favorite of all the roll variations! The savory nature of the bacon just seems to take the whole roll to a new flavor level I hadn't imagined before. Vegan bacon also works very well.

⅔ cup (80 grams) plain protein powder

3 cups flour

3 tablespoons sugar

2½ teaspoons baking powder

½ teaspoon baking soda

½ teaspoon salt

8 tablespoons butter or coconut oil

⅓ cup Greek yogurt

1 cup milk

1 egg

8 pieces crispy, cooked bacon, chopped into tiny pieces

¼ cup minced shallots

3 tablespoons liquid egg whites

2 teaspoons onion powder

1 teaspoon coarse salt

1 Preheat the oven to 425°F. Spray two or three baking sheets with cooking spray.

2 Combine the first six ingredients in a bowl or food processor. Chop the butter into tiny pieces and sprinkle them into the flour mixture, or drop the coconut oil in by the spoonful. Using the food processor or a pastry blender, combine the flour and butter/coconut oil until no more clumps remain.

3 In a large bowl, combine the mixture with the yogurt, milk, and egg with a spatula. You may need to use a stand mixer or your hands to fully combine all the ingredients, as it will be a somewhat dry dough.

4 Once the dough comes together, cut it into four equal pieces and place one section on a dry, clean surface. Flatten the dough, sprinkle it with one-fourth of the chopped bacon and shallots, and fold it over itself.

5 Press down, and repeat a few more times. Shape the dough into a square about ½-inch thick. Cut the square in half, and then use a knife to cut each rectangle into alternating triangles. Repeat the process with the remaining sections.

6 Place the triangles on the prepared baking sheet with some space around them. Brush the rolls with the egg whites and sprinkle with the onion powder and salt. Bake for 12 to 14 minutes, or until cooked through but still soft.

MAKES 25 ROLLS

NUTRITION PER ROLL				
119 calories	4 g fat	12 g carbs	12 g fiber	2 g protein

CRACKED PEPPER AND CHEDDAR ROLLS

Sometimes, you just need a little cheesy bread in your life. These rolls are the answer! But don't underestimate the cracked pepper in this recipe—it does wonders to complement the cheesy flavor.

⅔ cup (80 grams) plain protein powder

3 cups flour

3 tablespoons sugar

2½ teaspoons baking powder

½ teaspoon baking soda

½ teaspoon salt

8 tablespoons butter or coconut oil

⅓ cup Greek yogurt

1 cup milk

1 egg

½ cup shredded cheddar cheese

1 tablespoon cracked pepper

3 tablespoons liquid egg whites

1 teaspoon coarse salt

1 Preheat the oven to 425°F. Spray two or three baking sheets with cooking spray.

2 Combine the first six ingredients in a bowl or food processor. Chop the butter into tiny pieces and sprinkle them into the flour mixture, or drop the coconut oil in by the spoonful. Using the food processor or a pastry blender, combine the flour and butter/coconut oil until no more clumps remain.

3 In a large bowl, combine the mixture with the yogurt, milk, and egg with a spatula. You may need to use a stand mixer or your hands to fully combine all the ingredients, as it will be a somewhat dry dough.

4 Once the dough comes together, cut it into four equal pieces and place one section on a dry, clean surface. Flatten the dough, sprinkle it with one-fourth of the shredded cheese and pepper, and fold it over itself.

5 Press down, and repeat a few more times. Shape the dough into a square about ½-inch thick. Cut the square in half, and then use a knife to cut each rectangle into alternating triangles. Repeat the process with the remaining sections.

6 Place the triangles on the prepared baking sheet with some space around them. Brush the rolls with the egg whites and sprinkle with the salt. Bake 12 to 14 minutes, or until cooked through but still soft.

MAKES 25 ROLLS

NUTRITION PER ROLL				
117 calories	5 g fat	12 g carbs	2 g fiber	6 g protein

SPINACH DIJON ROLLS

*If you haven't included Dijon mustard in a roll recipe before, it's time you did.
I put it in on a whim and then could not get enough of the final product! I love
cutting them in half and filling them to make mini tea sandwiches.*

⅔ cup (80 grams) plain protein
  powder

3 cups flour

3 tablespoons sugar

2½ teaspoons baking powder

½ teaspoon baking soda

½ teaspoon salt

8 tablespoons butter or coconut oil

⅓ cup Greek yogurt

1 cup milk

1 egg

4 teaspoons Dijon mustard

½ cup chopped fresh spinach leaves

3 tablespoons liquid egg whites

1 teaspoon coarse salt

½ teaspoon garlic powder

1 Preheat the oven to 425°F. Spray two or three baking sheets with
  cooking spray.

2 Combine the first six ingredients in a bowl or food processor. Chop
  the butter into tiny pieces and sprinkle them into the flour mixture, or
  drop the coconut oil in by the spoonful. Using the food processor or
  a pastry blender, combine the flour and butter/coconut oil until no
  more clumps remain.

3 In a large bowl, combine the mixture with the yogurt, milk, and egg
  with a spatula. You may need to use a stand mixer or your hands to
  fully combine all the ingredients, as it will be a somewhat dry dough.

4 Once the dough comes together, cut it into four equal pieces and
  place one section on a dry, clean surface. Flatten the dough, spread
  on one-fourth of the Dijon mustard, sprinkle it with one-fourth of the
  chopped spinach, and fold it over itself.

5 Press down, and repeat a few more times. Shape the dough into
  a square about ½-inch thick. Cut the square in half, and then use
  a knife to cut each rectangle into alternating triangles. Repeat the
  process with the remaining sections.

6 Place the triangles on the prepared baking sheet with some space around them. Brush the rolls with the egg whites and sprinkle with the salt and garlic powder. Bake 12 to 14 minutes, or until cooked through but still soft.

MAKES 25 ROLLS

NUTRITION PER ROLL				
108 calories	4 g fat	12 g carbs	2 g fiber	5 g protein

SPINACH PARMESAN ROLLS

Thought spinach was just for salads? It is actually really perfect in these rolls, adding color and nutrition without taking anything away from the delicious and savory parmesan flavor.

½ cup (55 grams) plain protein powder

⅔ cup liquid egg whites

½ cup loosely packed spinach leaves, shredded

3 tablespoons shredded parmesan cheese (1 tablespoon reserved for topping)

1 tablespoon coconut oil, melted

2 tablespoon Greek yogurt

3 tablespoons ground flaxseed

½ teaspoon baking powder

½ teaspoon onion powder

½ teaspoon garlic powder

½ teaspoon ground white pepper

⅛ teaspoon salt

1 Preheat the oven to 400°F.

2 Mix all of the ingredients together in a large bowl.

3 Coat a muffin pan with baking spray. Portion the batter out evenly between eight of the muffin cups.

4 Sprinkle the 1 tablespoon of parmesan cheese among all the muffins.

5 Bake for about 12 minutes or just until the buns start to brown on the sides and look/feel fluffy. Allow to cool a few minutes before removing gently from the muffin tray.

MAKES 8 ROLLS | LOW-CARB | GLUTEN-FREE

NUTRITION PER ROLL				
100 calories	5 g fat	3 g carbs	2 g fiber	11 g protein

TORTILLAS/WRAPS

These super-easy wraps allow for great meal flexibility since you can make them quickly or even make ahead for some no-excuses healthy lunches. I like to fill them with anything from eggs to salads to peanut butter and jelly.

⅓ cup (40 grams) plain protein powder

⅓ cup flour

½ cup liquid egg whites

2 tablespoons coconut flour

1 tablespoon ground flaxseed

½ cup water

2 tablespoons oil

1 Preheat a nonstick pan coated in cooking spray over medium heat.

2 In a medium bowl, whisk all of the ingredients together to create a pasty batter. Pour a thin layer onto the preheated pan and cook through on one side before flipping to cook the other side.

3 Use immediately as a wrap or store for a day or two in the refrigerator. Reheat in a pan before using later.

MAKES 4 WRAPS

NUTRITION PER WRAP				
175 calories	8 g fat	11 g carbs	2 g fiber	14 g protein

SANDWICH BREAD

It's always nice not to feel guilty about eating bread! With all the protein and fiber in each serving, I know that I'm fueling my body and workouts the right way—even if I just want to snack on a plain slice of bread!

½ cup (55 grams) plain protein powder

2 cups flour

1½ teaspoons baking powder

½ teaspoon baking soda

1 teaspoon salt

¼ cup liquid egg whites

⅓ cup oil

1 cup water

1 Preheat the oven to 350°F. Coat a 9 x 5-inch loaf pan with cooking spray.

2 Combine the first five ingredients in a large bowl. Add in the remaining ingredients, and mix together thoroughly to combine. Scoop the dough into the prepared pan and place in the center rack of the preheated oven.

3 Bake about 45 minutes, or until browned on top and a toothpick inserted in the center comes out clean.

MAKES 12 SERVINGS

NUTRITION PER SERVING				
143 calories	7 g fat	14 g carbs	2 g fiber	8 g protein

CROUTONS

Once you've made the Sandwich Bread, the croutons are very simple to make. Add any seasonings you like and use them in salads and soups!

2 cups (or any amount) Sandwich Bread (page 114), cubed

garlic powder, salt, onion powder, and/or any desired seasonings

1 Preheat the oven to 400°F. Spray or oil a large baking sheet. Spread the cubed bread out evenly on top and spritz to coat with more oil.

2 Coat with an even layer of any desired seasonings and place in the center rack of the oven.

3 Bake about 15 minutes, or until browned and crunchy.

4 Store in a sealed bag at room temperature for a few days. If the croutons get stale, bake in the oven again for a few minutes right before using.

MAKES 4 SERVINGS

NUTRITION PER SERVING				
72 calories	3.5 g fat	7 g carbs	1 g fiber	4 g protein

PEANUT BUTTER SPREAD

With half the calories and the same amount of protein as regular peanut butter, I'd say this is a great alternative!

1 tablespoon (7 grams) vanilla or plain protein powder

2 ounces peanut butter

1 tablespoon water

2 teaspoons oil

Mix all of the ingredients together thoroughly to combine. Store, covered, in the refrigerator.

MAKES 3 SERVINGS | GLUTEN-FREE

NUTRITION PER SERVING				
109 calories	8 g fat	2 g carbs	1 g fiber	7 g protein

CREAM CHEESE SPREAD

Adding a little protein powder to your cream cheese is a super-easy way to make your meals or treats even more tasty and hunger satisfying!

2½ tablespoons (12 grams) vanilla or plain protein powder

2 ounces low-fat cream cheese

Mix the ingredients together thoroughly to combine. Store, covered, in the refrigerator.

MAKES 3 SERVINGS | GLUTEN-FREE

NUTRITION PER SERVING				
63 calories	4 g fat	2 g carbs	0 g fiber	6 g protein

WINTER SQUASH SOUP

This soup is wonderful for fall or winter, being at once a satisfying comfort food and a light, healthy meal. Baking the sweet potato and butternut squash can take some extra time, so prepare them ahead to make this dish even easier!

1 medium-small butternut squash

1 large or 2 small sweet potatoes (about 450 grams), skin on and scrubbed

1 (32-ounce) carton low-sodium chicken or vegetable broth

½ medium yellow onion

1 to 2 cloves garlic

small handful (about 6 to 8 small leaves) fresh sage

2 tablespoons extra virgin olive oil

½ teaspoon salt

¾ teaspoon ground pepper

¼ teaspoon cayenne pepper

¼ teaspoon garlic powder

¼ teaspoon onion powder

⅔ cup (80 grams) vanilla or plain protein powder

1 Preheat the oven to 375°F. Stab the butternut squash a few times through the middle and place on a baking sheet. Stick it in the oven for 20 minutes. Roll it over and bake for another 20 minutes. Repeat this once more to bake evenly through, until the squash is tender enough to be pierced with a fork. Remove from the oven and slice the squash in half lengthwise. Allow to cool enough to handle then peel and chop the squash.

2 Meanwhile, slice and discard any rough patches off the sweet potato. Chop the potato into large chunks, and place in a small, microwavable casserole dish. Pour enough of the broth over the sweet potato pieces to cover them about halfway and place a lid loosely on top. Microwave 8 to 10 minutes, or until all the chunks are fork-tender.

3 In a food processor, process the onion, garlic, and sage until almost smooth. Transfer to a small bowl and set aside.

4 Process the sweet potato and the squash in batches, using the broth from the sweet potato to help, until all of it is very smooth. Transfer to a large bowl and set aside.

5 Preheat a large stewpot over medium heat, then add the olive oil. When the oil is hot (but not smoking), add the onion mixture and sauté for 2 to 3 minutes before adding the blended sweet potato and squash. Add the rest of the broth, stopping short of the entire amount if you want a thicker consistency.

6 Add the salt, ground pepper, cayenne pepper, garlic powder, and onion powder and mix well. Bring the heat to a simmer and let everything come together for 10 to 15 minutes.

7 Take the soup off the heat. Using a whisk, stir the soup while you slowly add the protein powder. Continue to stir until it is well combined.

MAKES 8 SERVINGS | GLUTEN-FREE

NUTRITION PER SERVING				
140 calories	4 g fat	15 g carbs	3 g fiber	12 g protein

BROCCOLI CHEDDAR SOUP

This soup is great weeknight comfort food for winter. I love being able to eat something as nutritious as it is delicious, so I make this soup ahead of time to have once or twice more throughout the week!

4 cups chicken or vegetable stock

¼ large onion, diced

20 ounces frozen broccoli florets

3 cups fresh spinach

1½ cups shredded cheddar cheese

2 teaspoons garlic powder

1½ teaspoons paprika

1½ teaspoons white or black pepper

½ teaspoon salt, plus more, to taste

½ teaspoon cayenne pepper, or more, to taste

⅔ cup (80 grams) plain protein powder

1 In a large pot, bring the stock to a simmer. Add the onion and cook for about 5 minutes.

2 Add the next eight ingredients and simmer for about 3 more minutes, or until the frozen broccoli is just warmed through. Pour or ladle everything (carefully!) into a blender. Blend everything into a smooth consistency.

3 Take the soup off the heat. Using a whisk, stir the soup while you slowly add the protein powder. Continue to stir until it is well combined.

MAKES 8 SERVINGS | GLUTEN-FREE

NUTRITION PER SERVING				
91 calories	2 g fat	7 g carbs	2 g fiber	13 g protein

GRAVY

This is one of my absolute favorite recipes because the gravy tastes so delicious, and it is easily made vegan, gluten-free, and low-carb!

2 cups chicken or vegan "chicken" stock

½ teaspoon onion powder

½ teaspoon herb seasoning blend

pinch of salt

2 tablespoons oil

2 tablespoons (12 grams) plain protein powder

In a small saucepan, simmer the stock, onion powder, herb seasoning blend, and salt over high heat until reduced to ½ cup. Remove from heat and whisk in the oil, and then the protein powder, whisking as you add the powder so it doesn't curdle. Enjoy immediately or store, covered in the refrigerator, until ready to use.

MAKES 6 SERVINGS | LOW-CARB | GLUTEN-FREE

NUTRITION PER SERVING				
55 calories	5 g fat	0 g carbs	0 g fiber	3 g protein

QUICK HOMEMADE TOMATO SAUCE

I am a big fan of making my own tomato sauce, especially when it doesn't take all day! I can whip this up right along with dinner anytime. It's great to use on regular pasta, but for an extra helping of protein, try this on the Gnocchi (page 101) or the Pizza Crust (page 98).

1 (15-ounce) can diced tomatoes

½ (6-ounce) can tomato paste

¼ small yellow onion, chopped

2 cloves garlic, peeled

¼ cup packed fresh basil leaves

½ teaspoon ground white or black pepper

¼ teaspoon salt

¼ cup (30 grams) plain protein powder

1 Blend the first seven ingredients until the mixture is completely smooth. Heat a large saucepan over medium-high. When heated, add the tomato mixture and bring to a simmer. Allow to cook for 5 to 10 minutes to soften the flavors of the onion and garlic and to allow the ingredients to marry.

2 Remove from the heat and, stirring with a whisk, slowly add in the protein powder to incorporate it without curdling. Use on any pasta, pizza, or sandwich!

MAKES 8 SERVINGS | GLUTEN-FREE

NUTRITION PER SERVING				
51 calories	0 g fat	7 g carbs	1 g fiber	5 g protein

CANDY AND SWEET TREATS

If you're like me, you probably have a bit of a sweet tooth. With recipes like these, you can have your sweets, which are satisfying and give you an energy boost, without the crash or the guilt!

CHOCOLATE TRUFFLES

Believe me when I say that no one guesses that these are made with beans! The beans provide the structure and great texture, but any beany flavor is completely hidden behind the dark chocolate flavor. One of my very favorite treats to have around.

1 cup (110 grams) chocolate protein powder

1 (15-ounce) can black beans, rinsed and drained

½ cup ground flaxseed

2 tablespoons cocoa powder

¼ cup applesauce

½ cup agave syrup

½ cup stevia

⅓ cup cacao nibs or cocoa powder for finishing

FOR MINT CHOCOLATE TRUFFLES, ADD:

½ teaspoon mint extract

1 Process all of the ingredients together in a food processor (except the cacao nibs or cocoa powder) plus the mint extract, if using, until completely smooth.

2 Scoop the dough out into 1-inch portions and roll into balls.

3 Roll them in the cacao nibs or cocoa powder and enjoy! Store any extra in a sealed container in the refrigerator, or freeze.

MAKES 30 TRUFFLES | GLUTEN-FREE

NUTRITION PER TRUFFLE				
66 calories	2 g fat	10 g carbs	3 g fiber	7 g protein

PUMPKIN PIE TRUFFLES

These pumpkin pie truffles were a big hit with my cycling class when I brought them in! The fact that they are completely gluten-free and made with beans always blows people away.

⅔ cup (80 grams) vanilla or cinnamon protein powder

1 (15-ounce) can chickpeas, rinsed and drained

⅓ cup pumpkin puree

1½ cups oats

6 tablespoons flaxseed

½ cup agave syrup

¼ cup stevia

2 teaspoons vanilla extract

1 teaspoon ground cinnamon

1 teaspoon ground ginger

½ teaspoon nutmeg

¼ teaspoon allspice

3 graham crackers, crushed to crumbs, for finishing

1 Process all of the ingredients except the graham cracker crumbs together in a food processor until completely smooth.

2 Scoop the dough out into 1-inch portions and roll into balls.

3 Roll them in the graham cracker crumbs and enjoy! Store any extra in a sealed container in the refrigerator, or freeze.

MAKES 32 TRUFFLES | GLUTEN-FREE

NUTRITION PER TRUFFLE				
60 calories	1 g fat	10 g carbs	2 g fiber	7 g protein

LEMON DROP PROTEIN TRUFFLES

These are so tasty and soft and make the perfect treat right out of the refrigerator for any time. Sometimes, I'll grab a few for breakfast or one or two for a quick snack.

¾ cup (90 grams) lemon or vanilla protein powder

1 (15.9-ounce) can chickpeas, rinsed and drained

5 tablespoons agave syrup

½ cup ground flaxseed

1 large lemon, zested

¾ teaspoon lemon extract

¾ teaspoon salt

⅓ cup (40 grams) vanilla protein powder or oat flour, for finishing

1 Process all of the ingredients together in a food processor (except final ⅓ cup protein or oat flour) until completely smooth.

2 Scoop the dough out into 1-inch portions and roll into balls.

3 Roll them in the protein powder or oat flour and enjoy!

4 Store any extra in a sealed container in the refrigerator, or freeze.

MAKES 23 TRUFFLES | GLUTEN-FREE

NUTRITION PER TRUFFLE				
62 calories	1 g fat	8 g carbs	2 g fiber	7 g protein

PEANUT BUTTER AND JELLY BITES

If you didn't already know, I am a huge fan of peanut butter and jelly anything! These bites taste like tiny little sandwiches that are ready to go whenever I want a bit of PB and J! For the fresh berries, I use sliced strawberries, but feel free to substitute raspberries or another berry of your choosing.

⅓ cup (40 grams) vanilla, berry, or peanut butter protein powder

⅓ cup oats or ground flaxseed

½ cup peanut butter

½ cup oats

2 tablespoons agave syrup

1 tablespoon raspberry or strawberry jelly

¼ cup fresh berries

¼ teaspoon salt

1⅓ cups puffed millet

⅓ cup (40 grams) vanilla protein powder or oat flour, for finishing

1 Process all of the ingredients except the final ⅓ cup of vanilla protein powder or oat flour in a food processor until completely smooth.

2 Scoop the dough out into 1-inch portions and roll into balls.

3 Roll them in the protein powder or oat flour and enjoy! Store any extra in a sealed container in the refrigerator, or freeze.

MAKES 23 TRUFFLES | GLUTEN-FREE

NUTRITION PER SERVING				
70 calories	3 g fat	6 g carbs	1 g fiber	5 g protein

CHOCOLATE PEANUT BUTTER TRUFFLES

Peanut butter and chocolate go so well together, especially in this recipe. The peanut butter actually contributes wonderfully to the texture, making the truffles extra smooth.

⅔ cup (80 grams) chocolate protein powder

1 (15-ounce) can black beans, rinsed and drained

3 tablespoons cocoa powder

¼ teaspoon salt

⅓ cup peanut butter

¼ cup agave syrup

⅓ cup (40 grams) chocolate protein powder or cocoa powder, for finishing

1 Process all of the ingredients except the final ⅓ cup of chocolate protein powder or cocoa powder in a food processor until completely smooth.

2 Scoop the dough out into 1-inch portions and roll into balls.

3 Roll them in the protein powder or cocoa powder and enjoy! Store any extra in a sealed container in the refrigerator, or freeze.

MAKES 23 TRUFFLES | GLUTEN-FREE

NUTRITION PER TRUFFLE				
70 calories	2 g fat	7 g carbs	2 g fiber	6 g protein

BLACKBERRY ENERGY BITES

In the spring and summer when berries are at their freshest and most nutritious, I want to add them to just about everything! These energy bites take advantage of sweet, fresh blackberries or any variety of berry you like.

¾ cup (90 grams) vanilla protein powder1 (15-ounce) can chickpeas, rinsed and drained

⅔ cup fresh blackberries

2 tablespoons ground flaxseed

¼ teaspoon salt

⅓ cup stevia

⅓ cup sugar

1 teaspoon lemon extract

⅓ cup (40 grams) vanilla protein powder or oat flour for finishing

1 Process all of the ingredients except the final ⅓ cup of vanilla protein powder or oat flour in a food processor until completely smooth.

2 Scoop the dough out into 1-inch portions and roll into balls.

3 Roll them in the protein powder or oat flour and enjoy! Store any extra in a sealed container in the refrigerator, or freeze.

MAKES 23 TRUFFLES | GLUTEN-FREE

NUTRITION PER SERVING				
52 calories	0 g fat	8 g carbs	1 g fiber	6 g protein

HOMEMADE CHOCOLATE PEANUT CANDY BARS

Much better for you than a candy bar, this is the perfect recipe to make when you're in the mood for something sweet. It's very easy to make, and the result is absolutely delicious!

FOR THE CRUST:

⅓ cup (40 grams) vanilla protein powder

½ cup plus 2 tablespoons flour

¼ cup agave syrup

FOR THE NOUGAT:

¼ cup (30 grams) vanilla protein powder

¼ cup agave syrup

¼ cup unsweetened applesauce

1 egg

½ cup chopped roasted peanuts

For the chocolate coating:

2 tablespoons (12 grams) chocolate or vanilla protein powder

¼ cup coconut oil, melted

¼ cup cocoa powder

1 Preheat the oven to 350°F.

2 In a food processor, blend all of the ingredients for the crust together and press into the bottom of a greased 11 x 7-inch or 8 x 8-inch pan. Bake in the center of the oven for about 6 minutes or until just hardened.

3 Blend all of the nougat ingredients together except the peanuts. Pour evenly on top of the crust layer and spread the peanuts out across that. Bake another 5 minutes or so, to set.

4 Finally, blend all of the chocolate coating ingredients together and spread it evenly across the top of the nougat. Refrigerate for 1 hour, or until completely set. Cut into bars.

MAKES 16 BARS | GLUTEN-FREE

NUTRITION PER BAR				
113 calories	6 g fat	10 g carbs	1 g fiber	7 g protein

GUMMY BEARS

One of my favorite treats is fruity gummy candy. These are so easy to make that I'll prepare a huge batch and snack on them, guilt-free, all week! Try different fruit flavors like strawberry protein powder and strawberry—or orange-flavored gelatin.

3 tablespoons (20 grams) protein powder

½ cup water or juice

4 packets sugar-free, flavored gelatin

1 Mix all of the ingredients together in a metal bowl and set over a small pot with 1 inch of simmering water to make a double boiler. Use a whisk to stir as the gelatin dissolves.

2 Once the gelatin has completely dissolved, remove the bowl from the heat and spoon the mixture into silicone gummy bear (or any shape!) molds.

3 Place on a flat surface in the freezer for up to 10 minutes before removing to a sealed container. Store in the refrigerator.

MAKES ABOUT 15 GUMMIES | LOW-CARB | GLUTEN-FREE

NUTRITION PER GUMMY				
8 calories	0 g fat	0 g carbs	0 g fiber	2 g protein

GRILLED PEACHES WITH RICOTTA

Making treats with protein doesn't always have to be an involved process. One of the ways I like to use protein powder is mixed into a tasty cheese, like ricotta, and dolloped on a sweet, grilled peach. The result is always very satisfying!

2½ tablespoons (16 grams) vanilla protein powder

¼ cup low-fat ricotta cheese

1 large peach, halved

½ teaspoon ground cinnamon

1 Mix the vanilla protein powder and the ricotta together in a bowl.

2 Heat a grill or grill pan to medium-high heat. Spritz each peach half with oil, and grill for 4 to 5 minutes per side.

3 Place the peach, cut side up, on a plate, and dollop the ricotta onto each half. Sprinkle the cinnamon over the tops of each.

MAKES 1 SERVING | GLUTEN-FREE

NUTRITION PER SERVING				
217 calories	5 g fat	13 g carbs	2 g fiber	26 g protein

CHOCOLATE BARS

If you love a good chocolate bar with just the right amount of sweetness and a good snap to the bite, you can easily make your own—high in protein, healthy fat, antioxidants, and any other additions you might like—without all the added sugars and additives.

3 tablespoons (20 grams) chocolate protein powder

¼ cup coconut oil, melted

2 tablespoons cocoa powder

3 tablespoons stevia

1 to 2 tablespoons cacao nibs or other additions (optional)

1 Mix everything except the cacao nibs or other additions together very well.

2 Line an 8 x 5-inch pan with parchment paper, and pour the chocolate mixture into the pan. Spread out evenly and sprinkle on any additions that you like.

3 Freeze for about 15 minutes or until completely set. Transfer the chocolate bars to a sealed container and store in the refrigerator.

MAKES 4 LARGE SERVINGS | LOW-CARB | GLUTEN-FREE

NUTRITION PER SERVING				
181 calories	16 g fat	3 g carbs	3 g fiber	6 g protein

PUDDING AND ICE CREAM

It's easier than you think to make homemade protein pudding and ice cream—I love to do this and surprise my friends with it when they come to visit! All of these recipes are naturally healthier options for you, but if you'd like to reduce the sugar even more, feel free to swap out half or all of the sugar for another natural sweetener, such as erythritol or stevia.

CINNAMON BRÛLÉE
BREAD PUDDING

Whether you're looking for a really decadent dessert or just trying to use up some bread (try Sandwich Bread on page 114), these bread pudding recipes are some of the most scrumptious and easiest things you can ever make.

6 tablespoons (50 grams) vanilla or cinnamon protein powder

2 cups (about 56 grams) cubed bread

½ cup milk

2 ounces cream cheese or Cream Cheese Spread (page 117), softened

½ teaspoon ground cinnamon

¼ teaspoon nutmeg

1 tablespoon honey or sugar-free maple syrup (such as Walden Farms' calorie-free pancake syrup)

1 Toss all of the ingredients together and scoop into a small greased, oven-safe casserole dish or pan. For best results, cover and allow the bread to soak up the liquids for 4 hours or overnight in the refrigerator.

2 Preheat the oven to 350°F. Bake for 15 to 20 minutes or until the top is browned and the center of the pudding is still gooey.

MAKES 4 SERVINGS

NUTRITION PER SERVING				
135 calories	4 g fat	12 g carbs	2 g fiber	14 g protein

CARAMEL RAISIN BREAD PUDDING

6 tablespoons (50 grams) vanilla protein powder

2 cups (about 56 grams) cubed bread

½ cup milk

2 ounces cream cheese or Cream Cheese Spread (page 117), softened

½ teaspoon ground cinnamon

1 tablespoon caramel or sugar-free caramel syrup (such as Walden Farms' calorie-free pancake syrup)

¼ cup raisins

1 Toss all of the ingredients together and scoop into a small greased, oven-safe casserole dish or pan. For best results, cover and allow the bread to soak up the liquids for 4 hours or overnight in the refrigerator.

2 Preheat the oven to 350°F. Bake for 15 to 20 minutes or until the top is browned and the center of the pudding is still gooey.

MAKES 4 SERVINGS

NUTRITION PER SERVING				
165 calories	4 g fat	19 g carbs	2 g fiber	14 g protein

PEANUT BUTTER BREAD PUDDING

6 tablespoons (50 grams) vanilla or peanut butter protein powder

2 cups (56 grams) cubed bread

½ cup milk

3 tablespoons peanut butter or Peanut Butter Spread (page 116), softened

1 tablespoon honey or sugar-free caramel syrup (such as Walden Farms' calorie-free pancake syrup)

1 Toss all of the ingredients together and scoop into a small greased, oven-safe casserole dish or pan. For best results, cover and allow the bread to soak up the liquids for 4 hours or overnight in the refrigerator.

2 Preheat the oven to 350°F. Bake for 15 to 20 minutes or until the top is browned and the center of the pudding is still gooey.

MAKES 4 SERVINGS

NUTRITION PER SERVING				
144 calories	7 g fat	13 g carbs	2 g fiber	15 g protein

CHOCOLATE AVOCADO PUDDING

This is a rich and creamy pudding that works well for anyone avoiding dairy, and it tastes fabulous! Feel free to swap in banana slices for the strawberries.

⅓ cup (40 grams) chocolate protein powder

2 ripe avocados

⅓ cup chopped strawberries

2 tablespoons coconut oil

2 teaspoons vanilla extract

2 tablespoons cocoa powder

⅔ cup sugar

⅛ teaspoon salt

1 In a food processor, blend all of the ingredients.

2 Enjoy immediately, or store in the refrigerator in a sealed container for a few days.

MAKES 12 SERVINGS | GLUTEN-FREE

NUTRITION PER SERVING				
168 calories	6 g fat	26 g carbs	2 g fiber	3 g protein

PRO PUDDING

1 cup (110 grams) protein powder, any flavor

1 box sugar-free pudding mix, any flavor

2 cups milk

1 Blend all ingredients together for 3 to 5 minutes until very smooth and well combined.

2 Divide into cups and enjoy!

MAKES 3 SERVINGS | GLUTEN-FREE

NUTRITION PER SERVING				
140 calories	2 g fat	10 g carbs	1 g fiber	19 g protein

VANILLA ICE CREAM

These ice cream recipes really can be extremely easy to make and don't take a whole lot of time and effort. Plus, you'll have a much healthier version of your favorite frozen dessert that still tastes amazing! Try one of these ice creams in an Ice Cream Sandwich (page 196).

⅓ cup (40 grams) vanilla protein powder

⅓ cup almond milk

2 cups plain or vanilla Greek yogurt

¼ cup agave syrup

1 teaspoon vanilla extract *or* ½ teaspoon vanilla bean paste

1 Combine all of the ingredients and use with an ice cream maker according to its instructions.

2 OR combine all of the ingredients and spread into a thin layer in a large bowl and place in the freezer. Every 20 minutes, stir the ice cream together, spread thin, and replace in the freezer.

3 Repeat until the ice cream reaches the desired consistency and enjoy immediately, or store in a sealed container in the freezer.

4 To defrost, microwave for 10 seconds at a time until softened enough to stir together.

MAKES 4 SERVINGS | GLUTEN-FREE

NUTRITION PER SERVING				
176 calories	0 g fat	21 g carbs	0 g fiber	21 g protein

PUMPKIN ICE CREAM

⅓ cup (40 grams) pumpkin protein powder

1 cup Greek yogurt

¼ cup pumpkin puree

1 teaspoon pumpkin pie spice

1 teaspoon vanilla extract

3 tablespoons sugar

1 Combine all of the ingredients and use with an ice cream maker according to its instructions. Or combine the ingredients and spread into a thin layer in a large bowl and place in the freezer. Every 20 minutes, stir the ice cream together, spread thin, and replace in the freezer.

2 Repeat until the ice cream reaches the desired consistency and enjoy immediately, or store in a sealed container in the freezer.

3 To defrost, microwave for 10 seconds at a time until softened enough to stir together.

MAKES 4 SERVINGS | GLUTEN-FREE

NUTRITION PER SERVING				
133 calories	0 g fat	17 g carbs	0 g fiber	15 g protein

STRAWBERRY FROZEN YOGURT

¼ cup (30 grams) strawberry protein powder

1 cup Greek yogurt

2 tablespoons sugar-free strawberry jelly

⅔ cup chopped, fresh strawberries

2 tablespoons sugar

1 Combine all of the ingredients and use with an ice cream maker according to its instructions. Or combine the ingredients and spread into a thin layer in a large bowl and place in the freezer. Every 20 minutes, stir the ice cream together, spread thin, and replace in the freezer.

2 Repeat until the frozen yogurt reaches the desired consistency and enjoy immediately, or store in a sealed container in the freezer.

3 To defrost, microwave for 10 seconds at a time until softened enough to stir together.

MAKES 3 SERVINGS | GLUTEN-FREE

NUTRITION PER SERVING				
155 calories	0 g fat	17 g carbs	1 g fiber	20 g protein

MINT CHOCOLATE ICE CREAM

To make this wonderful, minty, green-tinted ice cream, I love to use spinach and fresh mint when I can. For the brownie chunks, use a homemade protein bar like the Fudgy Black Bean Brownies on page 209 or your favorite protein bar.

½ cup packed (10 grams) fresh mint leaves *or* ¼ teaspoon mint extract

½ cup packed (20 grams) fresh spinach *or* 2 drops green food coloring

⅓ cup milk

⅓ cup (40 grams) vanilla, mint, chocolate, or cookies-and-cream protein powder

2 cups Greek yogurt

¼ cup agave syrup

1 chocolate protein bar, chopped into pieces

1 If you are using the fresh mint leaves and the fresh spinach, process the leaves with the milk in a blender. Strain the liquid through a mesh colander into a medium bowl, extracting as much of the liquid as possible. Combine with all remaining ingredients and use with an ice cream maker according to its instructions.

2 If you are using the mint extract and green food coloring, combine all of the ingredients and spread into a thin layer in a large bowl and place in the freezer. Every 20 minutes, stir the ice cream together, spread thin, and replace in the freezer.

3 Repeat until the ice cream reaches the desired consistency and enjoy immediately, or store in a sealed container in the freezer.

4 To defrost, microwave for 10 seconds at a time until softened enough to stir together.

MAKES 4 SERVINGS | GLUTEN-FREE

NUTRITION PER SERVING				
175 calories	0 g fat	22 g carbs	0 g fiber	21 g protein

RASPBERRY BANANA SORBET

¼ cup (30 grams) vanilla or strawberry protein powder

1 large frozen ripe banana, sliced

½ cup frozen raspberries

1 In a food processor, blend all of the ingredients. If you need to, allow the ingredients to stand at room temperature up to 30 minutes until soft enough to blend.

2 Enjoy immediately, or store in the freezer in a sealed container. To defrost, microwave for 10 seconds at a time until softened enough to stir together.

MAKES 2 SERVINGS | GLUTEN-FREE

NUTRITION PER SERVING				
141 calories	0 g fat	22 g carbs	5 g fiber	14 g protein

BANANA ICE CREAM

¼ cup (30 grams) vanilla protein powder

2 large ripe frozen bananas, sliced

1 In a food processor, blend all of the ingredients. If you need to, allow the ingredients to stand at room temperature up to 30 minutes, until soft enough to blend.

2 Enjoy immediately, or store in the freezer in a sealed container. To defrost, microwave for 10 seconds at a time until softened enough to stir together.

MAKES 2 SERVINGS | GLUTEN-FREE

NUTRITION PER SERVING				
165 calories	0 g fat	30 g carbs	3 g fiber	14 g protein

FUDGY POPSICLES

½ cup (55 grams) chocolate protein powder

1 cup milk

1 tablespoon agave syrup

Blend all of the ingredients together and pour into Popsicle molds. Freeze until ready to eat!

MAKES 4 SERVINGS | GLUTEN-FREE

NUTRITION PER SERVING				
78 calories	1 g fat	5 g carbs	0 g fiber	13 g protein

STRAWBERRY PIE CREAMSICLES

1 recipe Strawberry Frozen Yogurt (page 142)

2 tablespoons strawberry jelly

1 graham cracker, crumbled

Blend all of the ingredients together and pour into Popsicle molds. Freeze until ready to eat!

MAKES 6 SERVINGS

NUTRITION PER SERVING				
97 calories	0 g fat	15 g carbs	0 g fiber	8 g protein

CUPCAKES, CAKES, AND FROSTINGS

You might think that healthy people avoid cake and frosting like the plague—but that doesn't have to be the case! Any of these make perfectly delicious celebratory treats, but unlike their store-bought counterparts, they're full of nutrients that will make your body happy, too!

This book would not be complete without the quintessential cupcake. Luckily, it's easy to make the perfect and healthy protein powder cupcake that's light, fluffy, and wonderful for any occasion! Pick a cupcake flavor, and then pair it with one of the frostings on pages 166–75.

VANILLA CUPCAKES

⅓ cup (40 grams) vanilla protein powder

½ cup applesauce

½ cup Greek yogurt

¼ cup oil

1 egg

½ cup sugar

½ cup stevia

1 tablespoon vinegar

2 teaspoons vanilla extract

1 cup flour

1 teaspoon baking powder

½ teaspoon baking soda

½ teaspoon salt

1 Preheat the oven to 350°F.

2 Combine the first nine ingredients in a large bowl. Add the remaining ingredients and mix well until just combined. Portion the batter out evenly into greased muffin cups.

3 Bake for 18 to 20 minutes or until just baked through, being careful not to overbake. Remove from the muffin pan and allow to cool completely on a wire rack.

MAKES 12 CUPCAKES

NUTRITION PER CUPCAKE				
138 calories	5 g fat	18 g carbs	1 g fiber	6 g protein

LEMON CHIA CUPCAKES

⅓ cup (40 grams) vanilla protein powder

⅓ cup applesauce

½ cup Greek yogurt

¼ cup oil

1 egg

½ cup sugar

½ cup stevia

2 tablespoons lemon juice

1 teaspoon lemon extract

1 cup flour

2 tablespoons whole chia seeds

1 teaspoon baking powder

½ teaspoon baking soda

½ teaspoon salt

1 Preheat the oven to 350°F.

2 Combine the first nine ingredients in a large bowl. Add the remaining ingredients and mix well until just combined. Portion the batter out evenly into greased muffin cups.

3 Bake for 18 to 20 minutes or until just baked through, being careful not to overbake. Remove from the muffin pan and allow to cool completely on a wire rack.

MAKES 12 CUPCAKES

NUTRITION PER CUPCAKE				
148 calories	6 g fat	18 g carbs	2 g fiber	6 g protein

CHOCOLATE-COVERED STRAWBERRY CUPCAKES

¼ cup (30 grams) chocolate protein powder

1 cup (222 grams) fresh strawberries, mashed

¾ cup butter, melted

¼ cup milk

¼ cup liquid egg whites

½ cup sugar

¼ cup stevia

1 teaspoon vanilla extract

2 cups flour

2 tablespoons cocoa powder

2 teaspoons baking powder

½ teaspoon salt

1 Preheat the oven to 350°F.

2 Combine the first eight ingredients in a large bowl. Add remaining ingredients and mix well until just combined. Portion the batter out evenly into greased muffin cups.

3 Bake for 18 to 20 minutes or until just baked through, being careful not to overbake. Remove from the muffin pan and allow to cool completely on a wire rack.

MAKES 12 CUPCAKES

NUTRITION PER CUPCAKE				
150 calories	5 g fat	21 g carbs	1 g fiber	6 g protein

CINNAMON SWIRL CUPCAKES

⅓ cup (40 grams) vanilla or cinnamon protein powder

½ cup applesauce

½ cup Greek yogurt

¼ cup oil

1 egg

½ cup sugar

½ cup stevia

1 tablespoon vinegar

2 teaspoons vanilla extract

1 cup flour

1 teaspoon cinnamon

1 teaspoon baking powder

½ teaspoon baking soda

½ teaspoon salt

FOR THE CINNAMON SWIRL:

¼ cup (30 grams) vanilla or cinnamon protein powder

3 tablespoons brown sugar

3 tablespoons applesauce

1½ teaspoons cinnamon

1 Preheat the oven to 350°F.

2 Combine the first nine ingredients in a large bowl. Add the remaining dry ingredients and mix well until just combined. Portion the batter out evenly into greased muffin cups.

3 Mix the cinnamon swirl ingredients together and portion it out in spoonfuls to swirl on top of each muffin.

4 Bake for 18 to 20 minutes or until just baked through, being careful not to overbake. Remove from the muffin pan and allow to cool completely on a wire rack.

MAKES 12 CUPCAKES

NUTRITION PER CUPCAKE				
150 calories	5 g fat	21 g carbs	1 g fiber	6 g protein

STRAWBERRY CUPCAKES

½ cup (55 grams) vanilla or strawberry protein powder

⅔ cup chopped fresh strawberries, pureed

⅓ cup Greek yogurt

¼ cup oil

1 egg

½ cup sugar

½ cup stevia

1 tablespoon vinegar

2 teaspoons vanilla extract

1¼ cups flour

1 teaspoon baking powder

½ teaspoon baking soda

½ teaspoon salt

1 Preheat the oven to 350°F.

2 Combine the first nine ingredients in a large bowl. Add the remaining ingredients and mix well until just combined. Portion the batter out evenly into greased muffin cups.

3 Bake for 18 to 20 minutes or until just baked through, being careful not to overbake. Remove from the muffin pan and allow to cool completely on a wire rack.

MAKES 12 CUPCAKES

NUTRITION PER CUPCAKE				
148 calories	5 g fat	18 g carbs	2 g fiber	7 g protein

CHOCOLATE CUPCAKES

½ cup (55 grams) vanilla protein powder

½ cup applesauce

½ cup Greek yogurt

¼ cup oil

1 egg

3 tablespoons cocoa powder

½ cup brown sugar

½ cup stevia

1 tablespoon vinegar

2 teaspoons vanilla extract

1 cup flour

1 teaspoon baking powder

½ teaspoon baking soda

½ teaspoon salt

1 Preheat the oven to 350°F.

2 Combine the first 10 ingredients in a large bowl. Add the remaining ingredients and mix well until just combined. Portion the batter out evenly into greased muffin cups.

3 Bake for 18 to 20 minutes or until just baked through, being careful not to overbake. Remove from the muffin pan and allow to cool completely on a wire rack.

MAKES 12 CUPCAKES

NUTRITION PER CUPCAKE				
138 calories	5 g fat	18 g carbs	1 g fiber	6 g protein

MARBLE CUPCAKES

1 recipe Vanilla Cupcakes (149)

1 recipe Chocolate Cupcakes (154)

1 Preheat the oven to 350°F.

2 Follow the directions for making the vanilla and chocolate cupcake batters. Pour the chocolate batter into two greased muffin pans, filling each cup only halfway. Pour the vanilla batter into the same cups. Use a knife to swirl the two batters together to create a marbled look.

3 Bake for 18 to 20 minutes or until just baked through, being careful not to overbake. Remove from the muffin pan and allow to cool completely on a wire rack.

MAKES 24 CUPCAKES

NUTRITION PER CUPCAKE				
138 calories	5 g fat	18 g carbs	1 g fiber	6 g protein

CHOCOLATE PEANUT BUTTER CUP CUPCAKES

1 recipe Chocolate Cupcakes (page 154)

FOR THE PEANUT BUTTER CUP FILLING:

¾ cup (90 grams) vanilla protein powder

6 tablespoons peanut butter

3 tablespoons agave syrup

4 tablespoons water

1 Preheat the oven to 350°F.

2 Prepare the chocolate cupcake batter. Pour *half* the batter into 12 greased muffin cups.

3 Mix all of the ingredients for the peanut butter cup filling and distribute evenly among all the cupcakes. Pour the remaining cupcake batter into all the muffin cups.

4 Bake for 18 to 20 minutes or until just baked through, being careful not to overbake. Remove from the muffin pan and allow to cool completely on a wire rack.

MAKES 12 CUPCAKES

NUTRITION PER CUPCAKE				
225 calories	9 g fat	23 g carbs	2 g fiber	13 g protein

BLACK FOREST CUPCAKES

1 recipe Chocolate Cupcakes (page 154)

1 cup pitted, drained cherries

1 Preheat the oven to 350°F.

2 Prepare the chocolate cupcake batter and mix in the cherries.

3 Pour the cupcake batter into 12 greased muffin cups.

4 Bake for 21 to 22 minutes or until just baked through, being careful not to over-bake. Remove from the muffin pan and allow to cool completely on a wire rack.

MAKES 12 CUPCAKES

NUTRITION PER SERVING				
163 calories	5 g fat	18 g carbs	2 g fiber	7 g protein

MINT CHOCOLATE CUPCAKES

1 recipe Chocolate Cupcakes (page 154)

½ cup peppermint or chocolate chips

¾ teaspoon peppermint extract

1 Preheat the oven to 350°F.

2 Prepare the chocolate cupcake batter and mix in the peppermint or chocolate chips and extract.

3 Pour the cupcake batter into 12 greased muffin cups.

4 Bake for 21 to 22 minutes or until just baked through, being careful not to overbake. Remove from the muffin pan and allow to cool completely on a wire rack.

MAKES 12 CUPCAKES

NUTRITION PER CUPCAKE				
193 calories	8 g fat	24 g carbs	2 g fiber	8 g protein

PUMPKIN SPICE LAYER CAKE

This recipe tastes like moist, yummy pumpkin cake, but is far lower in carbs and higher in protein than any other moist, yummy pumpkin cake!

¼ cup whole raw cashews

¼ cup (30 grams) vanilla, pumpkin, or cinnamon protein powder

⅓ cup tapioca flour

⅓ cup almond flour

1 teaspoon baking powder

½ teaspoon baking soda

1 cup packed pumpkin puree

4 eggs

½ cup melted butter or coconut oil

⅔ cup stevia

3 tablespoons ground flaxseed

1 teaspoon ground cinnamon

½ teaspoon allspice

½ teaspoon ground ginger

½ teaspoon nutmeg

Pumpkin Cream Cheese Frosting (page 173)

1 Preheat the oven to 350°F. Prep two 9-inch cake pans by greasing with coconut oil or spraying with baking spray.

2 Process the cashews in a food processor until they resemble a coarse meal. Then add in and blend all of the ingredients for the cake together in the food processor.

3 Divide the cake batter evenly between the two cake pans and bake for 30 to 35 minutes on the center rack until springy in the center and slightly browned. Place the pans on wire racks to cool for about 10 minutes before gently removing to fully cool on the rack.

4 In a blender or food processor, thoroughly combine all of the ingredients for the cream cheese frosting.

5 If the cake is cooled completely and the frosting is at room temperature, you can frost the tops of the cakes right away, and layer one on top of the other

6 Serve immediately or cover well and store in the refrigerator for up to a week.

MAKES 12 SLICES | LOW-CARB | GLUTEN-FREE

NUTRITION PER SLICE (without frosting)				
162 calories	13 g fat	7 g carbs	2 g fiber	6 g protein

FLOURLESS RHUBARB BLUEBERRY CAKE

This particular cake completely knocks my socks off. Beautifully purple, fluffy, and basically the most wonderful flourless cake ever, it makes a great dessert at parties—and it just happens to be low-carb!

1 (4-ounce) cup diced raw rhubarb

1 (5-ounce) cup fresh or frozen blueberries

1 cup butter or coconut oil

3 egg yolks

⅔ cup (80 grams) vanilla protein powder

2 tablespoons stevia

2 tablespoons white rum (optional)

1 teaspoon lemon extract

⅛ teaspoon salt

3 tablespoons liquid egg whites at room temperature

⅛ teaspoon cream of tartar

1 Preheat the oven to 375°F.

2 In a small saucepan, simmer the rhubarb and blueberries about 10 minutes to make a thick jam. Blend in a blender until smooth.

3 Combine the coconut oil and butter with the jam, whisking until the oil and butter is completely incorporated with the jam. Set aside to cool slightly, about 5 minutes.

4 In a small bowl, combine the egg yolks, protein powder, stevia, white rum (if using), lemon extract, and salt, and whisk until just blended. Pour the yolk mixture over the cooled butter mixture and whisk until no streaks of egg are visible.

5 In a stand mixer or a large, clean mixing bowl, combine the egg whites and cream of tartar. Use the whip attachment and beat until stiff peaks are created.

6 Using a rubber spatula, gently fold in the egg whites with the rhubarb blueberry mixture until no white streaks remain.

7 Pour the batter into a greased springform pan and smooth the top. Bake until the cake looks almost firm, but still jiggles slightly when moved, for 20 to 23 minutes.

8 Transfer to a wire rack and let cool in the pan for 30 minutes. The cake will sink slightly in the middle. Run a thin knife along the inside edge of the pan to loosen the cake, then release the sides and lift them off.

9 Let the cake cool completely for about 1 hour more before covering and storing in the refrigerator or cutting and serving.

MAKES 16 SERVINGS | LOW-CARB | GLUTEN-FREE

NUTRITION PER SERVING (without crust)				
148 calories	13 g fat	2 g carbs	0 g fiber	6 g protein

GINGER POUND CAKE

The soft density of this pound cake is what makes it stand out among cakes. The addition of ginger (or cinnamon, if you prefer) and your choice of fruit puree takes this pound cake to new levels as well!

½ cup Cashew Cream Frosting (page 167)

½ cup (55 grams) vanilla protein powder

¾ cup (7 ounces) any fruit puree

1½ teaspoons ground ginger

½ cup milk

½ cup sugar

½ cup stevia

1 tablespoon vinegar

1 teaspoon vanilla extract

1¾ cups flour

1½ teaspoons baking powder

½ teaspoon salt

1 Preheat the oven to 325°F.

2 Thoroughly combine the Cashew Cream Frosting with the eight ingredients that follow. Mix in the flour, baking powder, and salt.

3 Scoop the batter into two greased 8 x 4-inch loaf pans or one 8 x 8-inch baking pan, and bake for about 35 minutes, or until just done.

4 Allow to cool for at least 10 minutes in the pan before running a knife around the edges and removing, or leave in the pan and store, covered, at room temperature for up to 2 days. Alternatively, freeze in a freezer-safe bag or store in a sealed container in the refrigerator for up to a week.

MAKES 12 SLICES

NUTRITION PER SLICE				
229 calories	5 g fat	40 g carbs	3 g fiber	6 g protein

VANILLA SPONGE CAKE

This soft sponge cake is great for making thin, square layer cakes or simply for frosting and rolling up into a jelly roll–style cake!

⅓ cup (40 grams) vanilla protein powder

3 eggs

2 tablespoons coconut oil

1 teaspoon vanilla extract

¼ cup sugar

½ cup flour

¾ teaspoon baking powder

1 Preheat the oven to 350°F.

2 Thoroughly combine the first five ingredients. Add the flour and baking powder and mix well to combine.

3 Pour into a greased 13 x 9-inch pan and bake for 15 to 20 minutes or until just baked through.

MAKES 12 SLICES

NUTRITION PER SLICE				
103 calories	4 g fat	12 g carbs	1 g fiber	5 g protein

MARBLE LAYER CAKE

I wouldn't trade any boxed mix for this light and fluffy marble cake—it's almost too good to be true!

½ cup (55 grams) vanilla protein powder

⅓ cup applesauce

⅓ cup oil

1 cup sugar

⅔ cup milk

3 eggs

1 tablespoon vanilla extract

2 cups flour

1½ teaspoons baking powder

½ teaspoon baking soda

½ teaspoon salt

2 tablespoons cocoa powder

1 Preheat the oven to 350°F.

2 Combine the first seven ingredients in a large bowl. Add the remaining dry ingredients, minus the cocoa powder, to the bowl, mixing well until just combined.

3 Portion *half* the batter out evenly into two greased cake pans.

4 Add the cocoa powder to the remaining cake batter and scoop into each of the cake pans by the spoonful. Use a knife to swirl the chocolate and vanilla batters together.

5 Bake for about 25 minutes or until just baked through, being careful not to overbake. Cool for a few minutes before carefully removing from the cake pans, and allow to cool completely on a wire rack.

6 Frost with the Chocolate Cream Cheese Frosting (page 171).

MAKES 12 SLICES

NUTRITION PER SLICE (without frosting)				
314 calories	8 g fat	49 g carbs	3 g fiber	13 g protein

RED VELVET SHEET CAKE

The velvety-soft texture and chocolatey taste of this cake doesn't belie anything different about it. No one ever guesses that it's made with heart-healthy and workout-boosting beets!

1 cup (110 grams) chocolate protein powder

1 (15-ounce) can whole or sliced beets, with packing water

1 egg

¼ cup oil

1¼ cups sugar

⅓ cup cocoa powder

1⅓ cups flour

1½ teaspoons baking powder

½ teaspoon baking soda

½ teaspoon salt

1 Preheat the oven to 350°F.

2 Combine the first six ingredients in a food processor. Add the remaining ingredients and mix or pulse in the food processor until just combined. Pour the batter into a greased 12 x 9-inch pan.

3 Place in the oven for about 35 minutes or until just cooked through, being careful not to overbake. Cool completely before slicing to serve or frosting.

MAKES 16 SLICES

NUTRITION PER SLICE (without frosting)				
165 calories	0 g fat	30 g carbs	3 g fiber	14 g protein

CHOCOLATE AVOCADO FROSTING

It may seem like an unlikely base for a frosting, but the creaminess of the avocado perfectly replaces butter in this recipe for a lower calorie, higher-nutrition frosting that tastes as good as any other chocolate buttercream frosting!

⅓ cup (40 grams) chocolate protein powder

2 ripe Hass avocados

¼ cup coconut oil

1 teaspoon vanilla extract

2 tablespoons cocoa powder

⅔ cup sugar

1 In a food processor or blender, combine all of the ingredients completely. Use immediately, or store for a few days in a sealed container in the refrigerator.

MAKES ABOUT 16 SERVINGS | GLUTEN-FREE

NUTRITION PER SERVING				
140 calories	6 g fat	19 g carbs	1 g fiber	3 g protein

Tip: For Mocha Frosting, add 2 tablespoons instant coffee or espresso powder.

CASHEW CREAM FROSTING

The flavor of raw cashews mimics the flavor and texture of creamy cheese so well that it's a common ingredient in many vegan or dairy-free recipes. Definitely worth a try if you haven't yet!

1 cup raw cashews

½ cup (55 grams) vanilla protein powder

1 teaspoon vanilla extract

⅓ cup powdered sugar

6 tablespoons milk

1 For the best results, soak cashews in water for 4 hours or overnight, and drain before using.

2 In a food processor or blender, combine all of the ingredients completely. Use immediately, or store for a few days in a sealed container in the refrigerator.

MAKES ABOUT 10 SERVINGS | GLUTEN-FREE

NUTRITION PER SERVING				
117 calories	5 g fat	11 g carbs	0 g fiber	7 g protein

VANILLA SILK FROSTING

In this recipe, tofu adds a creamy texture with few calories for its high-protein content. This frosting is very easy to make vegan or dairy-free—just be sure to refrigerate it!

¾ cup raw cashews

1 scoop (30 grams) vanilla protein powder

½ (12-ounce) package extra-firm silken tofu (such as Mori-Nu)

¼ cup sugar

1 teaspoon vanilla extract

1 For best results, soak cashews in water for 4 hours or overnight, and drain before using.

2 In a food processor or blender, combine all of the ingredients completely. Use immediately, or store for a few days in a sealed container in the refrigerator.

MAKES ABOUT 10 SERVINGS | GLUTEN-FREE

NUTRITION PER SERVING				
84 calories	4 g fat	6 g carbs	0 g fiber	5 g protein

CREAM CHEESE FROSTING

This frosting is delicious on almost anything, from cakes to cookies, just like a traditional cream cheese frosting. Feel free to use a low-fat cream cheese and/or stevia or agave instead of sugar.

⅓ cup (40 grams) vanilla protein powder

1 (8-ounce) package cream cheese

⅓ cup sugar

½ teaspoon vanilla extract

1 In a food processor or blender, combine all of the ingredients completely. Use immediately, or store for a few days in a sealed container in the refrigerator.

MAKES ABOUT 10 SERVINGS | GLUTEN-FREE

NUTRITION PER SERVING				
101 calories	4 g fat	9 g carbs	0 g fiber	6 g protein

STRAWBERRY CREAM CHEESE FROSTING

Fresh strawberries make a very delicious and natural frosting—much better than buying one with artificial flavors and food colorings.

⅓ cup (40 grams) vanilla or strawberry protein powder

1 (8-ounce) package low-fat cream cheese

⅔ cup chopped fresh strawberries

⅓ cup sugar/sweetener

½ teaspoon vanilla extract

1 In a food processor or blender, combine all of the ingredients completely. Use immediately, or store for a few days in a sealed container in the refrigerator.

MAKES ABOUT 12 SERVINGS | GLUTEN-FREE

NUTRITION PER SERVING				
86 calories	4 g fat	8 g carbs	0 g fiber	5 g protein

CHOCOLATE CREAM CHEESE FROSTING

Use this one instead of the other cream cheese or chocolate frostings, or swirl it in with strawberry or vanilla frosting for a marbled look!

⅓ cup (40 grams) chocolate protein powder

1 (8-ounce) package low-fat cream cheese

⅓ cup sugar

1 tablespoon cocoa powder

1 teaspoon vanilla extract

1 In a food processor or blender, combine all of the ingredients completely. Use immediately, or store for a few days in a sealed container in the refrigerator.

MAKES ABOUT 10 SERVINGS | GLUTEN-FREE

NUTRITION PER SERVING				
101 calories	4 g fat	9 g carbs	0 g fiber	6 g protein

CINNAMON CREAM CHEESE FROSTING

This is THE frosting to use on top of the Cinnamon Swirl Cupcakes (page 152) or in the Cinnamon Brûlée or Caramel Raisin Bread Pudding recipes (pages 135 and 136)!

⅓ cup (40 grams) vanilla or cinnamon protein powder

1 (8-ounce) package low-fat cream cheese

⅓ cup sugar

1 teaspoon ground cinnamon

1 teaspoon vanilla extract

In a food processor or blender, combine all of the ingredients completely. Use immediately, or store for a few days in a sealed container in the refrigerator.

MAKES ABOUT 10 SERVINGS | GLUTEN-FREE

NUTRITION PER SERVING				
101 calories	4 g fat	9 g carbs	0 g fiber	6 g protein

PUMPKIN CREAM CHEESE FROSTING

For a little taste of fall, you can put this frosting on any cookie, cupcake, or cake! I especially love to use this with the Pumpkin Spice Layer Cake (page 159).

¼ cup (30 grams) vanilla or cinnamon protein powder

⅓ cup (50 grams) pumpkin puree

½ cup (4 ounces) full-fat cream cheese

⅓ cup stevia

½ teaspoon ground cinnamon

1 In a food processor or blender, combine all of the ingredients completely. Use immediately, or store for a few days in a sealed container in the refrigerator.

MAKES ABOUT 10 SERVINGS | LOW-CARB | GLUTEN-FREE

NUTRITION PER SERVING				
56 calories	4 g fat	1 g carbs	0 g fiber	4 g protein

LEMONY MANGO FROSTING

This frosting is beautifully lemon-yellow, but it is colored and made primarily with ripe mango! The mango flavor takes a backseat to the lemon but adds sweetness and a creamy body to the frosting. Great with the Vanilla Sponge Cake (page 163)!

½ cup (55 grams) vanilla protein powder

1 cup chopped fresh mango

⅔ cup powdered sugar

1 teaspoon lemon extract

1 tablespoon coconut oil

¼ teaspoon salt

In a food processor or blender, combine all of the ingredients completely. Use immediately, or store for a few days in a sealed container in the refrigerator.

MAKES ABOUT 10 SERVINGS | GLUTEN-FREE

NUTRITION PER SERVING				
79 calories	2 g fat	11 g carbs	0 g fiber	5 g protein

BERRY FROSTING

Made mostly with fresh berries (I like using strawberries and/or blackberries), this is one of the most guilt-free frostings I've ever had. Still, when people try this one, they can't believe it's actually so much better for you than regular frosting

¾ cup (90 grams) vanilla protein powder

1 cup fresh berries

⅓ cup agave syrup

1 teaspoon lemon extract

⅛ teaspoon salt

In a food processor or blender, combine all of the ingredients completely. Use immediately, or store for a few days in a sealed container in the refrigerator.

MAKES ABOUT 10 SERVINGS | GLUTEN-FREE

NUTRITION PER SERVING				
74 calories	0 g fat	11 g carbs	0 g fiber	8 g protein

COOKIES AND PIES

From weekday afternoon snacks to desserts worth sharing with company, these surprisingly healthy recipes are crowd-pleasers that will definitely satisfy your sweet tooth!

In addition, this section includes some of the best combinations of cookies and frostings. Try one of them out, and feel free to get creative.

MOCHA SNICKERDOODLES

This latte-inspired spin on snickerdoodles works well with the cinnamon-sugar coating!

¼ cup (30 grams) chocolate protein powder

1 cup flour

2 teaspoons instant coffee or espresso powder

1 teaspoon baking soda

¼ teaspoon cream of tartar

⅛ teaspoon salt

1 egg

1 tablespoon melted coconut oil

2 teaspoons vanilla extract

½ cup Greek yogurt

½ cup applesauce

¼ cup brown sugar

3 tablespoons sugar

1 tablespoon cinnamon

1 Preheat the oven to 350°F. Coat two baking sheets with cooking spray.

2 In a large bowl, whisk the first six ingredients together. Mix in the next six ingredients to combine.

3 In a small bowl, combine the remaining sugar and cinnamon. Drop the cookie dough by rounded tablespoons into the sugar and cinnamon, rolling it around to coat.

4 Place the cookies 1½ inches apart on the baking sheet.

5 Bake in the oven for 9 to 10 minutes or until just baked through. They will finish setting as they cool.

MAKES 25 COOKIES

NUTRITION PER COOKIE				
43 calories	1 g fat	7 g carbs	1 g fiber	3 g protein

STRAWBERRY LEMONADE COOKIES

Strawberry lemonade in a cookie? Yes, please!

¼ cup (30 grams) strawberry protein powder

1½ cups flour

⅓ cup oats

1 teaspoon baking soda

¼ teaspoon salt

½ cup sugar

1 large lemon, zested

⅓ cup lemon juice

¼ cup cold butter, chopped

1 cup chopped fresh strawberries

½ teaspoon lemon extract

1 Preheat the oven to 350°F. Coat two baking sheets with cooking spray.

2 Blend all of the ingredients together in a food processor just until completely combined.

3 Scoop the batter into 1½ to 2-inch round scoops and place on the cookie sheets with about 2 inches of space in between each one.

4 Bake for 10 to 13 minutes or until just baked through. Allow to cool for about 2 minutes before transferring to a cooling rack.

MAKES 15 COOKIES

NUTRITION PER COOKIE				
111 calories	3 g fat	17 g carbs	2 g fiber	3 g protein

CHOCOLATE SANDWICH COOKIES

These homemade and healthy cookies are so much fun to present to someone that it's definitely worth the bit of extra effort to make them!

FOR THE FILLING:

¼ cup (30 grams) vanilla protein powder

1 (4-ounce) package cream cheese at room temperature

FOR THE COOKIES:

1 scoop (35 grams) chocolate protein powder

½ cup dried cherries

2 tablespoons cocoa powder

2 tablespoons coconut oil

½ cup raw almonds or cashews

2 tablespoons ground flaxseed

½ cup oats

1 Preheat the oven to 350°F. Coat a baking sheet with cooking spray.

2 Make the filling. In a small bowl, combine the vanilla protein powder and cream cheese.

3 Make the cookies. Blend all of the ingredients together in a food processor until completely combined.

4 Scoop the batter into 1-inch round scoops and press into circles, evenly spaced, on the cookie sheets.

5 Bake for 8 to 9 minutes or until just baked through.

6 Allow to cool before frosting and pressing the cookies together. Store in an airtight container in the refrigerator or freeze.

MAKES ABOUT 23 SANDWICH COOKIES | GLUTEN-FREE

NUTRITION PER SANDWICH COOKIE				
94 calories	4 g fat	12 g carbs	2 g fiber	4 g protein

LEMON SUGAR COOKIES

Perfect for cutting out into shapes and frosting, these are extra fun for special occasions.

1 (12-ounce) package extra-firm silken tofu

⅓ cup (40 grams) vanilla protein powder

½ cup lemon juice

1 lemon, zested

½ cup brown sugar

½ cup sugar

1 teaspoon lemon extract

⅓ cup applesauce

2 tablespoons ground flaxseed

2 cups flour

1½ teaspoons baking powder

½ teaspoon baking soda

¼ teaspoon salt

FOR THE FROSTING:

1 recipe Vanilla Silk Frosting (page 168)

½ teaspoon lemon extract

1 lemon, zested

1 Preheat the oven to 350°F. Coat two baking sheets with cooking spray.

2 Blend one-half of the tofu with the remaining cookie ingredients in a food processor just until completely combined. (You will use the remaining half of the tofu package for the Vanilla Silk Frosting.)

3 Dust a smooth, clean, dry surface with flour and scoop the dough on top. Dust the dough with more flour to avoid sticking, and roll out to about ¼ inch thick. Use a cookie cutter to cut out cookies and space them out evenly on the baking sheet.

4 Bake for 10 to 13 minutes or until just baked through. Allow to cool for about 2 minutes before transferring to a cooling rack.

5 Meanwhile, prepare the frosting. Frost just before serving.

MAKES ABOUT 25 COOKIES

NUTRITION PER COOKIE				
83 calories	1 g fat	17 g carbs	1 g fiber	4 g protein

CHOCOLATE CHIP COOKIES

For when you just need an old-fashioned chocolate chip cookie!

¼ cup (30 grams) vanilla protein powder

1 cup flour

1 teaspoon baking powder

¼ teaspoon salt

¼ cup applesauce

¼ cup liquid egg whites

¼ cup coconut oil

½ teaspoon vanilla extract

1 cup sugar

3 tablespoons mini chocolate chips

1 Preheat the oven to 350°F. Coat two baking sheets with cooking spray.

2 Mix all of the ingredients together just until completely combined. Scoop the batter into 1½- to 2-inch round scoops and place on the cookie sheets with about 2 inches of space in between each one.

3 Bake for about 8 minutes or until just baked through. Allow to cool for about 2 minutes before transferring to a cooling rack.

MAKES ABOUT 16 COOKIES

NUTRITION PER COOKIE				
137 calories	4 g fat	22 g carbs	1 g fiber	3 g protein

OATMEAL RAISIN COOKIES

One of my very favorite cookies growing up, this recipe is one I'll always come back to. Here it's made much better for a healthy lifestyle!

½ cup (55 grams) vanilla or cinnamon protein powder

1 cup oats

⅔ cup flour

1 teaspoon baking soda

½ teaspoon ground cinnamon

¼ teaspoon nutmeg

¼ teaspoon salt

⅓ cup applesauce

¼ cup butter or coconut oil

¼ cup liquid egg whites

⅓ cup brown sugar

⅓ cup sugar

½ teaspoon vanilla extract

1 Preheat the oven to 350°F. Coat two baking sheets with cooking spray.

2 Mix all of the ingredients together just until completely combined. Scoop the batter into 1½- to 2-inch round scoops and place on the cookie sheets with about 2 inches of space in between each one.

3 Bake for about 8 minutes or until just baked through. Allow to cool for about 2 minutes before transferring to a cooling rack.

MAKES ABOUT 16 COOKIES

NUTRITION PER COOKIE				
164 calories	3 g fat	18 g carbs	1 g fiber	8 g protein

CHOCOLATE CAKE COOKIES

Don't look now… but cake and cookies have made a baby! These cookies really taste and feel like cake but are just right for a cookie-sized snack.

⅓ cup (40 grams) chocolate protein powder

1 cup flour

⅓ cup cocoa powder

¾ teaspoon baking powder

½ teaspoon baking soda

¼ teaspoon salt

¼ cup liquid egg whites

1 egg

⅓ cup Greek yogurt

¼ cup coconut oil

¼ cup agave syrup

1 teaspoon vanilla extract

1 Preheat the oven to 350°F. Coat two baking sheets with cooking spray.

2 Mix all of the ingredients together just until completely combined. Scoop the batter into 1½- to 2-inch round scoops and place on the cookie sheets with about 2 inches of space in between each one.

3 Bake for about 11 minutes or until just baked through. Allow to cool for about 2 minutes before transferring to a cooling rack.

MAKES ABOUT 16 COOKIES

NUTRITION PER COOKIE				
88 calories	4 g fat	11 g carbs	2 g fiber	3 g protein

FLOURLESS PEANUT BUTTER COOKIES

Nope, there really is no flour in these cookies! (Even after you try them, you might still not believe it.)

⅓ cup (40 grams) vanilla or peanut butter protein powder

½ cup ground flaxseed

¼ teaspoon baking powder

¼ teaspoon salt

⅔ cup milk

⅓ cup peanut butter

½ teaspoon vanilla extract

2 tablespoons butter or coconut oil, melted

⅓ cup brown sugar

¼ cup sugar

1 egg

¼ cup liquid egg whites

1 Preheat the oven to 350°F. Coat two baking sheets with cooking spray.

2 Mix all of the ingredients together just until completely combined. Scoop the batter into 1½- to 2-inch round scoops and place on the cookie sheets with about 2 inches of space in between each one.

3 Bake for 12 to 14 minutes or until just baked through. Allow to cool for about 2 minutes before transferring to a cooling rack.

MAKES ABOUT 12 COOKIES | GLUTEN-FREE

NUTRITION PER COOKIE				
130 calories	6 g fat	14 g carbs	2 g fiber	7 g protein

FLOURLESS ALMOND APRICOT COOKIES

⅓ cup (40 grams) vanilla protein powder

½ cup ground flaxseed

¼ teaspoon baking powder

¼ teaspoon salt

⅔ cup milk

⅓ cup almond butter

¼ teaspoon almond extract

2 tablespoons butter or coconut oil, melted

⅓ cup brown sugar

¼ cup sugar

1 egg

¼ cup liquid egg whites

⅓ cup chopped dried apricots

1 Preheat the oven to 350°F. Coat two baking sheets with cooking spray.

2 Mix all of the ingredients together just until completely combined. Scoop the batter into 1½- to 2-inch round scoops and place on the cookie sheets with about 2 inches of space in between each one.

3 Bake for 12 to 14 minutes or until just baked through. Allow to cool for about 2 minutes before transferring to a cooling rack.

MAKES ABOUT 12 COOKIES | GLUTEN-FREE

NUTRITION PER COOKIE				
140 calories	6 g fat	16 g carbs	2 g fiber	7 g protein

GREEN TEA COOKIES

Matcha green tea is great in so much more than drinks! It adds flavor and antioxidants to these cookies. You can find matcha powder online or at health food stores.

¼ cup (30 grams) vanilla protein powder

1 cup flour

2 tablespoons matcha green tea powder

1 teaspoon baking soda

¼ teaspoon cream of tartar

⅛ teaspoon salt

1 egg

1 tablespoon melted coconut oil

2 teaspoons vanilla extract

½ cup Greek yogurt

½ cup applesauce

¼ cup plus 3 tablespoons sugar, divided

1 Preheat the oven to 350°F. Coat two baking sheets with cooking spray.

2 In a large bowl, whisk together the first six ingredients. Mix in the next five ingredients, plus the ¼ cup sugar to combine.

3 Drop the cookie dough by rounded tablespoons into the remaining 3 tablespoons of sugar, and roll it around to coat. Place the cookies 1½ inches apart on the baking sheet.

4 Bake in the oven for 9 to 10 minutes or until just baked through. They will finish setting as they cool.

MAKES 25 COOKIES

NUTRITION PER COOKIE				
53 calories	1 g fat	7 g carbs	1 g fiber	3 g protein

VANILLA BREAKFAST COOKIES

With all their healthy, nutritious ingredients, I like to think of these as cookies you could even eat for breakfast. I often do! If you need a gluten-free cookie, just be sure to buy gluten-free certified oats.

1½ cups plus 2 cups rolled oats, divided

⅓ cup (40 grams) vanilla protein powder

6 Medjool dates, pitted

6 dried apricots

½ cup liquid egg whites

3 ounces (about 6 tablespoons) pureed avocado

2 tablespoons stevia

6 tablespoons Greek yogurt

¼ cup stevia

1 Preheat the oven to 350°F. Coat three cookie sheets with cooking spray.

2 Blend 1½ cups of the rolled outs with all of the remaining ingredients in a food processor.

3 Scoop the batter into a large bowl and mix in the remaining 2 cups of rolled oats.

4 Use a small scoop to portion out rounded 1½ tablespoons of batter across the cookie sheets.

5 Bake for 10 to 12 minutes or until golden brown on top and soft but cooked in the middle. Cool and enjoy!

MAKES 35 COOKIES | GLUTEN-FREE

NUTRITION PER COOKIE				
56 calories	1 g fat	10 g carbs	1 g fiber	3 g protein

GIANT CHOCOLATE BREAKFAST COOKIES

3½ cups rolled oats, separated

6 Medjool dates, pitted

6 dried apricots

½ cup liquid egg whites

6 tablespoons pureed avocado

2 tablespoons stevia

⅓ cup (40 grams) chocolate protein powder

½ cup Greek yogurt

¼ cup stevia

2 heaping tablespoons cocoa powder

1 Preheat the oven to 350°F. Coat three cookie sheets with cooking spray.

2 Blend 1½ cups of the rolled oats with the remaining ingredients in a food processor.

3 Scoop the batter into a large bowl and mix in the remaining 2 cups of rolled oats.

4 Use a small scoop to portion out rounded 1½ tablespoons of batter across the cookie sheets.

5 Bake for 10 to 12 minutes or until golden brown on top and soft but cooked in the middle. Cool and enjoy!

MAKES 13 COOKIES | GLUTEN-FREE

NUTRITION PER COOKIE				
141 calories	3 g fat	7 g carbs	3 g fiber	24 g protein

CRUNCHY PECAN COOKIES

Sometimes I like to have crunchier cookies that I can dunk in milk or tea, and these are just right for that. I love the tasty pecan and slight coconut flavors.

¼ cup (30 grams) vanilla protein powder

⅓ cup almond flour

2 tablespoons ground flaxseed

2 tablespoons ground chia seeds

2 tablespoons sweetened dried coconut shreds

2 tablespoons finely crushed pecans

¼ teaspoon cream of tartar

¾ teaspoon baking soda

⅛ teaspoon salt

¼ cup liquid egg whites

3 tablespoons coconut oil

6 tablespoons stevia

1 tablespoon water, if needed, to moisten dough

1 Preheat the oven to 350°F. Coat two baking sheets with cooking spray.

2 Mix the first nine ingredients together in one bowl.

3 Mix the egg whites, coconut oil, and stevia in another bowl.

4 Blend the wet ingredients with the dry until it forms a thick batter, and add the 1 tablespoon water if needed to bind the ingredients better.

5 Divide into 16 round balls, and place onto the baking sheets.

6 Bake for 12 to 13 minutes or until semi-firm, but not hard. Cool on a wire rack, and enjoy!

MAKES 16 COOKIES | LOW-CARB | GLUTEN-FREE

NUTRITION PER COOKIE				
75 calories	5½ g fat	4 g carbs	1 g fiber	3 g protein

PEANUT BUTTER AND JELLY THUMBPRINTS

Tiny, crunchy peanut butter cookies with a jelly center couldn't be any cuter! Using stevia and sugar-free jelly keeps them low-carb, but feel free to use real sugar if you prefer.

⅓ cup (40 grams) vanilla or peanut butter protein powder

⅔ cup almond flour

¼ cup coconut flour

¾ teaspoon baking soda

¼ teaspoon salt

¼ cup ground flaxseed

2 tablespoons coconut oil, melted

½ cup softened or room temperature peanut butter

2 eggs

½ cup stevia

sugar-free raspberry jelly

1 Preheat the oven to 350°F. Coat a baking sheet with cooking spray. Mix the first five ingredients together in one medium bowl.

2 Combine the next five ingredients in another bowl, mixing well before adding them to the dry mixture until they are well combined.

3 Drop tablespoon-sized balls, evenly spaced, onto the baking sheet. Press down to flatten into thick discs and make a well in the center of each one by pressing with a finger.

4 Fill the centers with a little jelly, and bake the cookies on the center rack of the oven for about 6 minutes or until just baked through and barely crunchy.

5 Cool on a wire rack, and enjoy!

MAKES 50 COOKIES | LOW-CARB | GLUTEN-FREE

NUTRITION PER COOKIE				
39 calories	3 g fat	2 g carbs	1 g fiber	2 g protein

PUMPKIN BUTTER COOKIES

These cookies are delicious on their own; or, take them to another level as a sandwich with Pumpkin Cream Cheese Frosting (page 173) or Pumpkin Ice Cream (page 141).

¼ cup (30 grams) vanilla protein powder

1 cup flour

1 teaspoon baking soda

¼ teaspoon cream of tartar

⅛ teaspoon salt

1 egg

1 tablespoon melted coconut oil

2 teaspoons vanilla extract

½ cup Greek yogurt

½ cup pumpkin puree

¼ cup brown sugar

1 tablespoon, plus ¾ teaspoon cinnamon, divided

½ teaspoon ground ginger

½ teaspoon allspice

¼ teaspoon nutmeg

3 tablespoons sugar

1 Preheat the oven to 350°F. Coat two baking sheets with cooking spray.

2 In a large bowl, whisk the first five ingredients together. Mix in the remaining ingredients, except for the sugar and the ¾ teaspoon of cinnamon.

3 In a small bowl, combine the remaining sugar and cinnamon. Drop the cookie dough by rounded tablespoons into the sugar and cinnamon, and roll it around to coat. Place the cookies 1½ inches apart on the baking sheet.

4 Bake in the oven for 9 to 10 minutes or until just baked through. They will finish setting as they cool.

MAKES 25 COOKIES

NUTRITION PER COOKIE				
48 calories	1 g fat	7 g carbs	2 g fiber	3 g protein

SPICED MOLASSES COOKIES

Right around Christmas time, I start to crave those warm flavors of spices and molasses. These are great with either vanilla or chocolate protein powder.

⅓ cup (40 grams) vanilla or chocolate protein powder

1 cup flour

¾ teaspoon baking powder

½ teaspoon baking soda

¼ teaspoon salt

¼ cup liquid egg whites

1 egg

⅓ cup Greek yogurt

¼ cup coconut oil

¼ cup molasses

1 teaspoon vanilla extract

½ teaspoon ground cinnamon

½ teaspoon ground ginger

¼ teaspoon cloves

1 Preheat the oven to 350°F. Coat two baking sheets with cooking spray.

2 Mix all of the ingredients together just until completely combined.

3 Scoop the batter into 1½- to 2-inch round scoops and place on the cookie sheets with about 2 inches of space in between each one.

4 Bake for about 11 minutes or until just baked through. Allow to cool for about 2 minutes before transferring to a cooling rack.

MAKES 25 COOKIES

NUTRITION PER COOKIE				
55 calories	1 g fat	8 g carbs	1 g fiber	3 g protein

LEMONY LAYER SANDWICHES

1 recipe Lemon Sugar Cookies (page 180)

1 recipe Lemony Mango Frosting (page 174)

1 Prepare the Lemon Sugar Cookies and the Lemony Mango Frosting according to the recipe instructions. When the cookies have completely cooled, frost the bottom of one cookie, and press the bottom of another cookie into it to form a sandwich.

2 Serve immediately or store in an airtight container in the refrigerator for a few days.

NUTRITION PER SANDWICH (2 cookies and ½ serving frosting)				
205 calories	2 g fat	39 g carbs	3 g fiber	10 g protein

CHOCOLATE-COVERED BERRY SANDWICHES

1 recipe Chocolate Cake Cookies (page 183)

1 recipe Berry Frosting (page 175)

1 Prepare the Chocolate Cake Cookies and the Berry Frosting according to the recipe instructions. When the cookies have completely cooled, frost the bottom of one cookie, and press the bottom of another cookie into it to form a sandwich.

2 Serve immediately or store in an airtight container in the refrigerator for a few days.

NUTRITION PER SANDWICH (2 cookies and ½ serving frosting)				
214 calories	8 g fat	28 g carbs	3 g fiber	11 g protein

PUMPKIN PIE SANDWICHES

1 recipe Pumpkin Butter Cookies (page 191)

1 recipe Pumpkin Cream Cheese Frosting (page 173)

1 Prepare the Pumpkin Butter Cookies and the Pumpkin Cream Cheese Frosting according to the recipe instructions. When the cookies have completely cooled, frost the bottom of one cookie, and press the bottom of another cookie into it to form a sandwich.

2 Serve immediately or store in an airtight container in the refrigerator for a few days.

NUTRITION PER SANDWICH (2 cookies and ½ serving frosting)				
128 calories	3 g fat	16 g carbs	2 g fiber	7 g protein

ICE CREAM SANDWICHES

If cookies are great on their own, they're even better with ice cream sandwiched between them! Try any cookie recipe from pages 177–92 with any ice cream recipe from pages 140–45.

    1 recipe for any cookie

    1 recipe for any ice cream

1 Prepare the cookies and the ice cream.

2 Allow the ice cream to sit at room temperature for 10 to 20 minutes or until softened to a consistency you can scoop.

3 When the cookies have completely cooled, place one scoop of ice cream on top of a cookie and press another cookie into it to make a sandwich.

4 Enjoy immediately or store in an airtight container in the freezer until ready to enjoy!

NUTRITION PER SANDWICH (2 Strawberry Lemonade cookies and ½ serving Vanilla Ice Cream)*				
312 calories	7 g fat	44 g carbs	4 g fiber	18 g protein

* This will change depending on cookie and ice cream

CHEESECAKE

It can be tough to find a satisfying cheesecake that isn't over the top in fat and sugar, but this recipe is just rich, creamy, and sweet enough to make the perfect dessert—without giving you a toothache—or stomachache!

FOR THE CRUST:

1 recipe Vanilla Cookie Pie Crust (page 204) or Nut-Free Chocolate Crust (page 203)

FOR THE FILLING:

¼ cup (30 grams) vanilla protein powder

8 ounces reduced-fat cream cheese

½ cup Greek yogurt

¼ teaspoon salt

¼ cup agave syrup

⅓ cup stevia

1 tablespoon cornstarch or tapioca flour or arrowroot powder

1 teaspoon vanilla extract

1 Preheat the oven to 350°F.

2 Prepare and bake the Vanilla Cookie or Nut-Free Chocolate Pie Crust recipe in a springform pan.

3 Combine all of the filling ingredients in a mixer or blender. Scoop the entire filling onto the crust.

4 Bake for about 25 minutes until set. Cool to room temperature, then store in the refrigerator until ready to serve.

MAKES 8 SLICES

NUTRITION PER SLICE (WITHOUT CRUST)				
122 calories	5 g fat	11 g carbs	0 g fiber	8 g protein

PUMPKIN PIE CHEESECAKE

If you like pumpkin pie and you like cheesecake, just think how much better your life will be with this protein-packed, healthier Pumpkin Pie Cheesecake!

FOR THE CRUST:

¾ cup almond flour

¾ cup ground flaxseed

4 tablespoons butter or coconut oil

⅛ teaspoon salt

FOR THE CHEESECAKE FILLING:

8 ounces reduced-fat cream cheese

3 eggs

2 tablespoons liquid egg whites

1 teaspoon vanilla extract

¼ cup tapioca flour, arrowroot powder, or cornstarch

6 ounces yogurt

½ cup stevia

FOR THE PUMPKIN PIE FILLING:

½ cup (55 grams) vanilla protein powder

2 cups pumpkin puree

¾ cup milk

3 tablespoons tapioca flour, arrowroot powder, or cornstarch

⅔ cup stevia

1 teaspoon ground cinnamon

½ teaspoon ground ginger

½ teaspoon allspice

¼ to ½ teaspoon nutmeg

1 Preheat the oven to 350°F.

2 In a food processor or mixing bowl, combine all of the ingredients for the crust. Press the dough down into a thin layer on two greased 8 x 8-inch square baking sheets or two 8-inch or 9-inch round pie pans. Bake the crust for 6 to 8 minutes, or until it seems just done.

3 Blend all of the ingredients for the cheesecake filling in a food processor or mixer and set aside. Separately, do the same for the pumpkin pie filling.

4 Distribute the cheesecake filling evenly between the two baked pie crusts. Then, scoop out the pumpkin pie filling, using a spoon to scoop it into different places throughout the cheesecake filling. Use a knife to gently swirl the cheesecake and the pumpkin pie filling together.

5 Bake the cheesecakes on the center rack for about 50 minutes. The cheesecake should be moist but not too wet when it's done.

6 Chill about 2 hours before enjoying.

MAKES 32 DECADENT SQUARES OR SLICES

NUTRITION PER SLICE				
88 calories	6 g fat	5 g carbs	1 g fiber	3 g protein

PUMPKIN PIE

As soon as the first whiff of fall is in the air, I start craving pumpkin everything! My best answer to those cravings is my famous pumpkin pie—and yes, this has been gobbled up at several of my Thanksgiving and Christmas dinners in the past.

FOR THE CRUST:

>   1 recipe Vanilla Cookie Pie Crust
>   (page 204)

FOR THE FILLING:

>   ½ cup (55 grams) vanilla, pumpkin, chocolate, or cinnamon protein powder
>
>   1 cup Greek yogurt
>
>   1 (15-ounce) can pumpkin puree
>
>   1 teaspoon ground cinnamon
>
>   ½ teaspoon ground ginger
>
>   ½ teaspoon allspice
>
>   ¼ teaspoon nutmeg
>
>   ⅓ cup stevia powder
>
>   2 tablespoons vanilla extract

1 Preheat the oven to 350°F.

2 Prepare and bake the Vanilla Cookie Pie Crust or other crust recipe in a springform pan.

3 Combine all of the ingredients in a mixer or blender. Scoop the entire filling onto the crust.

4 Bake for about 30 minutes until set. Cool to room temperature, then store in the refrigerator until ready to serve

MAKES 8 SLICES | GLUTEN-FREE

NUTRITION PER SLICE (without pie crust)				
67 calories	0 g fat	6 g carbs	1 g fiber	10 g protein

CHOCOLATE CREAM PIE

This is definitely one of my all-time favorite ways to eat chocolate—in pie form! Not only is it easy to make, it looks and tastes really impressive!

FOR THE CRUST:

1 recipe Chocolate Cashew Pie Crust (page 203)

FOR THE FILLING:

8 ounces reduced-fat cream cheese

8 ounces Greek yogurt

½ cup (55 grams) chocolate protein powder

¼ teaspoon salt

⅓ cup stevia

⅓ cup agave syrup

2 tablespoons vanilla extract

¼ cup cocoa powder

1 Preheat the oven to 350°F.

2 Prepare and bake the Chocolate Cashew Pie Crust recipe in a springform pan.

3 In a mixer or blender, combine all of the ingredients. Scoop the entire filling onto the crust.

4 Bake about 30 minutes until set. Cool to room temperature, then store in the refrigerator until serving.

MAKES 8 SLICES | GLUTEN-FREE

NUTRITION PER SLICE (without pie crust)				
154 calories	5 g fat	11 g carbs	0 g fiber	12 g protein

MARGARITA PIE

This is a pie for your next celebratory affair! It tastes seriously delicious—like a margarita mixed with ice cream and made into a pie—and it will make everyone happy, from your healthy eaters to your decadent dessert lovers!

FOR THE CRUST:

9 graham crackers

1 tablespoon agave syrup

2 tablespoons fresh lemon or lime juice

FOR THE FILLING:

¾ cup (90 grams) vanilla or lemon protein powder

1 (12.3-ounce) block extra-firm tofu (such as Mori-Nu)

2 limes, zested

2 teaspoons lemon extract

¼ teaspoon salt

½ cup Greek yogurt

3 tablespoons sugar-free margarita mix or lime juice

⅓ cup powdered sugar or stevia

¼ cup agave syrup

2 tablespoons tequila (optional)

1 Preheat the oven to 350°F.

2 Combine all of the ingredients for crust in a food processor. Press the dough into the bottom of a greased pie pan. Bake the crust for about 7 minutes to harden.

3 In a mixer or blender, combine all ingredients for the filling. Scoop the entire filling into the prepared crust.

4 Bake the pie for about 20 minutes. Cool to room temperature, then store in the refrigerator until ready to serve.

MAKES 8 SLICES

NUTRITION PER SLICE (WITHOUT CRUST)				
150 calories	1 g fat	18 g carbs	1 g fiber	9 g protein

PIE CRUSTS

Personally, fussing over finicky pie crusts is not how I like to spend my time. All of these crusts are extremely easy to make and can be mixed and matched with any of the pie fillings on pages 200–201!

NUT-FREE CHOCOLATE PIE CRUST

⅓ cup (40 grams) chocolate protein powder

½ cup oats

1 tablespoon cocoa powder

3 tablespoons ground flaxseed

¼ teaspoon salt

3 tablespoons agave syrup

1 tablespoon water

1 Preheat the oven to 350°F.

2 Blend all of the ingredients together in a food processor. Press the dough into the bottom of a greased pie pan, and bake for about 8 minutes.

MAKES 8 SERVINGS | GLUTEN-FREE

NUTRITION PER SERVING				
78 calories	2 g fat	11 g carbs	2 g fiber	6 g protein

CHOCOLATE CASHEW PIE CRUST

¼ cup (30 grams) chocolate protein powder

1 cup cashews

¼ cup ground flaxseed

2 tablespoons coffee or milk

1 tablespoon agave syrup

1 Preheat the oven to 350°F.

2 Blend all of the ingredients together in a food processor. Press the dough into the bottom of a greased pie pan, and bake for about 7 minutes.

MAKES 8 SERVINGS | GLUTEN-FREE

NUTRITION PER SERVING				
111 calories	6 g fat	9 g carbs	2 g fiber	6 g protein

VANILLA COOKIE PIE CRUST

¼ cup (30 grams) vanilla protein powder

¾ cup cashews or almonds

6 tablespoons ground flaxseed

2 tablespoons Greek yogurt or applesauce

1 tablespoon agave syrup

1 Preheat the oven to 350°F.

2 Blend all of the ingredients together in a food processor. Press the dough into the bottom of a greased pie pan, and bake for about 6 minutes.

MAKES 8 SERVINGS | GLUTEN-FREE

NUTRITION PER SERVING				
112 calories	7 g fat	7 g carbs	2 g fiber	6 g protein

BARS AND BROWNIES

Why buy lots of expensive protein bars with ingredients you can't pronounce when you can bake one at home that tastes even better? This chapter is full of some of the most dessert-like protein bars ever— but you can still take them with you on the go! Don't be afraid to wrap them individually and pop them in the freezer or refrigerator for a convenient snack.

RED VELVET BROWNIES

The beets bring out a natural reddish tint to these dense, chocolatey brownies, but they also give them a velvety, moist texture and heart-healthy nutrients!

1 (15-ounce) can whole or sliced beets, drained

⅔ cup (80 grams) chocolate protein powder

2 tablespoons oil

1¼ cups sugar

¼ cup cocoa powder

1 cup flour

¾ teaspoon baking powder

½ teaspoon baking soda

½ teaspoon salt

1 Preheat the oven to 350°F.

2 Drain the beets and combine them with the next four ingredients in a food processor until no lumps remain. Add the remaining ingredients and mix or pulse in the food processor until just combined. Pour the batter into a greased 12 x 9-inch or 8 x 8-inch pan.

3 Bake for about 35 minutes in the 12 x 9-inch pan or 45 minutes in the 8 x 8-inch pan until just baked through, being careful not to overbake. Cool completely before slicing to serve or frosting.

MAKES 16 BROWNIES

NUTRITION PER BROWNIE				
131 calories	2 g fat	24 g carbs	2 g fiber	6 g protein

CHOCOLATE STRAWBERRY CHEESECAKE BROWNIES

When I combined these two recipes, imagining I would get some kind of cheesecake swirl brownie, I instead found that, when almost completely mixed together, they make an even better cakelike brownie!

1 recipe Chocolate Cake Cookies (page 183)

½ recipe Strawberry Cream Cheese Frosting (page 170)

1 Preheat the oven to 350°F.

2 Prepare the Chocolate Cake Cookie dough, then prepare the Strawberry Cream Cheese Frosting. Thoroughly combine all but ¼ cup of the prepared frosting with the Chocolate Cake Cookie dough.

3 Pour the batter into a greased 8 x 8-inch pan and smooth the top. Swirl the remaining frosting into the top of the batter.

4 Bake 20 to 25 minutes or until baked through but still soft. Cool completely before slicing to serve or frosting.

MAKES 12 BROWNIES

NUTRITION PER BROWNIE				
160 calories	4 g fat	19 g carbs	1 g fiber	6 g protein

PEANUT BUTTER BROWNIE BARS

For the peanut butter and chocolate lovers out there…this one's for you.

heaping ½ cup (70 grams) chocolate protein powder

1 cup flour

3 tablespoons cocoa powder

¾ teaspoon baking powder

½ teaspoon baking soda

½ teaspoon salt

2 tablespoons ground flaxseed

⅔ cup liquid egg whites

½ cup peanut butter

⅓ cup sugar

1 Preheat the oven to 350°F.

2 Combine the first seven ingredients in a large bowl. Add the egg whites, peanut butter, and sugar, and mix well to combine.

3 Pour the batter into a greased 8 x 8-inch pan and smooth the top.

4 Bake for about 25 to 30 minutes until just baked through, being careful not to overbake. Cool completely before slicing to serve.

MAKES 12 BROWNIE BARS

NUTRITION PER BAR				
156 calories	6 g fat	16 g carbs	3 g fiber	11 g protein

FUDGY BLACK BEAN BROWNIES

If you haven't yet tried a black bean brownie, start with this one. It will completely change your perspective on beans—you wouldn't know they were in the brownies if you didn't put them in yourself!

½ cup (55 grams) chocolate protein powder

1 (15-ounce) can black beans, rinsed and drained

¼ cup cocoa powder

¼ cup coconut oil

¼ cup applesauce

⅓ cup brown sugar

⅓ cup stevia

3 tablespoons ground flaxseed

1 teaspoon vanilla extract

¾ teaspoon baking soda

½ teaspoon salt

1 Preheat the oven to 350°F.

2 Blend all of the ingredients together in a food processor until smooth and scoop into a greased 8 x 8-inch pan.

3 Bake on the center rack for about 30 minutes. The center will still be soft but not gooey.

4 Allow to cool completely before cutting into bars and serving.

MAKES 16 BROWNIES | GLUTEN-FREE

NUTRITION PER BROWNIE				
98 calories	4 g fat	10 g carbs	2 g fiber	5 g protein

CHICKPEA BIRTHDAY CAKE BARS

Shh…don't tell the other recipes, but this one might be my favorite! Not only is it extremely easy to make, but with a good vanilla protein powder, it really does have a very birthday cake flavor. It also impresses everyone to find out that they are made with chickpeas!

½ cup (55 grams) vanilla protein powder

1 (15-ounce) can chickpeas, rinsed and drained

½ cup raw cashews

¼ cup coconut oil

¼ cup applesauce

⅓ cup brown sugar

⅓ cup stevia

3 tablespoons ground flaxseed

1 teaspoon vanilla extract

¾ teaspoon baking soda

½ teaspoon salt

rainbow sprinkles, to top

1 Preheat the oven to 350°F.

2 Blend all of the ingredients together in a food processor until smooth and scoop into a greased 8 x 8-inch pan.

3 Sprinkle on the rainbow sprinkles. Bake on the center rack for about 30 minutes. The center will still be soft but not gooey.

4 Allow to cool completely before cutting into bars and serving.

MAKES 16 BARS | GLUTEN-FREE

NUTRITION PER COOKIE				
141 calories	6 g fat	11 g carbs	2 g fiber	5 g protein

BANANA BUTTERSCOTCH BAKED OATMEAL

Very tasty Banana Butterscotch Baked Oatmeal bars are a great way to make breakfast to grab and go for the week. If you or a family member needs them to be gluten-free, just be sure to buy gluten-free certified oats.

½ cup (55 grams) vanilla protein powder

2 large bananas

¼ cup agave syrup

½ cup stevia

⅓ cup liquid egg whites

2 tablespoons coconut oil

1 teaspoon maple flavor or vanilla extract

1½ cups oats or oat flour

1 teaspoon baking soda

½ teaspoon salt

1½ cups oats

¼ cup butterscotch chips, plus 2 tablespoons for topping

1 Preheat the oven to 350°F.

2 Combine the first eight ingredients in a food processor or large bowl, mixing well until no lumps remain.

3 Mix in the remaining ingredients, minus the 2 tablespoons of butterscotch chips.

4 Pour the batter into a greased 8 x 11-inch pan and smooth the top. Sprinkle the last 2 tablespoons of butterscotch chips on top.

5 Bake for about 30 minutes until just baked through, being careful not to overbake.

6 Cool completely before slicing to serve.

MAKES 16 SERVINGS | GLUTEN-FREE

NUTRITION PER SERVING				
156 calories	4 g fat	20 g carbs	2 g fiber	10 g protein

BERRY BAKED OATMEAL

Made with LOTS of antioxidant and fiber-packed berries, these baked oatmeal bars are a great way to make breakfast to grab and go for the week. If you or a family member needs them to be gluten-free, just be sure to buy gluten-free certified oats.

½ cup (55 grams) vanilla or cinnamon protein powder

2 (10-ounce) cups fresh or frozen and thawed berries

½ cup stevia

⅓ cup liquid egg whites

2 tablespoons coconut oil

1½ cups oats or oat flour

1 teaspoon baking soda

½ teaspoon salt

1½ cups oats

1 Preheat the oven to 350°F.

2 Combine the first six ingredients in a food processor until no lumps remain.

3 Mix in the baking soda, salt, and oats. Pour the batter into a greased 8 x 11-inch pan and smooth the top.

4 Bake for about 30 minutes until just baked through, being careful not to overbake.

5 Cool completely before slicing to serve.

MAKES 16 FUDGE BROWNIES | GLUTEN-FREE

NUTRITION PER COOKIE				
149 calories	4 g fat	18 g carbs	2 g fiber	10 g protein

FUDGY CARROT CAKE PROTEIN BARS

Fudge and carrot cake walked into a protein bar … well, when you try these, you'll know it was a good idea!

1 cup chopped carrots

⅔ cup pitted dates

¼ cup raw cashews

1 cup (110 grams) vanilla or cinnamon protein powder

½ cup (4 ounces) reduced fat cream cheese

¾ cup ground flaxseed

1 tablespoon coconut oil

1 (15-ounce) can chickpeas, rinsed and drained

⅓ cup stevia in the raw

2 teaspoons pumpkin pie spice

1 Preheat the oven to 350°F.

2 Blend the carrots, dates, and cashews together in a food processor until smooth.

3 Add in the remaining ingredients and blend again until smooth.

4 Scoop the dough into a greased 11 x 7-inch or 8 x 8-inch pan.

5 Bake on the center rack for 25 to 30 minutes. The center will still be soft but not gooey.

6 Allow to cool completely before cutting into bars and serving.

MAKES 20 SERVINGS | GLUTEN-FREE

NUTRITION PER SERVING				
105 calories	5 g fat	9 g carbs	3 g fiber	8 g protein

GRANOLA BARS

Granola bars make wonderful snacks, but the prepackaged kind at the grocery store usually have so many ingredients you don't want and little to no protein! These will keep you full longer, and you can add anything you like to make them delicious!

½ cup (55 grams) vanilla protein powder

3 cups rolled oats

½ cup ground flaxseed

⅓ cup coconut or almond flour

1 cup applesauce

½ cup honey

¼ cup oil

¼ teaspoon salt

Optional additions: coconut flakes, chocolate chips, nuts, chia seeds, dried fruit, etc.

1 Preheat the oven to 350°F.

2 Combine all of the ingredients together in a mixing bowl.

3 Scoop the batter into a greased 13 x 9-inch pan and press down on the top to create a thin, dense layer.

4 Bake for 25 to 30 minutes. Cool completely before slicing to serve.

MAKES 20 BARS | GLUTEN-FREE

NUTRITION PER BAR				
135 calories	5 g fat	18 g carbs	3 g fiber	5 g protein

Tip: For crunchier granola bars, place the sliced bars on a pan and bake for another 5 to 10 minutes.

PUFFED MILLET CRISPY TREATS

If you like Rice Krispies Treats, you'll love these. They are even better for you and your family, made with blood-sugar-stabilizing protein, healthy coconut oil, and whole millet.

20 large marshmallows

¼ cup coconut oil

¼ cup (30 grams) vanilla protein powder

2⅔ cups puffed millet

1 Coat a 8 x 8-inch pan with cooking spray.

2 Melt the marshmallows with coconut oil in a large, microwave-safe bowl on medium heat or in a large pot over the stove over medium heat, just until melted, taking care not to burn the marshmallows.

3 Mix in the vanilla protein powder and then the puffed millet. Before it hardens, press the crispy treat mass into the greased pan.

4 Allow to set at room temperature before slicing to serve.

MAKES 12 SERVINGS | GLUTEN-FREE

NUTRITION PER SERVING				
109 calories	5 g fat	12 g carbs	0 g fiber	3 g protein

CONVERSIONS

Temperature Conversions

FAHRENHEIT (°F)	CELSIUS (°C)
325°F	165°C
350°F	175°C
375°F	190°C
400°F	200°C
425°F	220°C
450°F	230°C

Volume Conversions

U.S.	U.S. EQUIVALENT	METRIC
1 tablespoon (3 teaspoons)	½ fluid ounce	15 milliliters
¼ cup	2 fluid ounces	60 milliliters
⅓ cup	3 fluid ounces	90 milliliters
½ cup	4 fluid ounces	120 milliliters
⅔ cup	5 fluid ounces	150 milliliters
¾ cup	6 fluid ounces	180 milliliters
1 cup	8 fluid ounces	240 milliliters
2 cups	16 fluid ounces	480 milliliters

Weight Conversions

U.S.	METRIC
½ ounce	15 grams
1 ounce	30 grams
2 ounces	60 grams
¼ pound	115 grams
⅓ pound	150 grams
½ pound	225 grams
¾ pound	350 grams
1 pound	450 grams

RECIPE INDEX

ABOUT THE AUTHOR

Courtney K. Nielsen is a fitness professional and a healthy recipe and lifestyle blogger from Arizona. She is an AFAA-certified personal trainer and group fitness instructor and has been creating healthy and delicious recipes for her blog, FitCakes, at FitCakery.com since 2011. When she isn't developing new recipes, she loves to teach indoor cycling classes, challenge herself to lift heavier weights at the gym, write, and cook for her friends and family.